The Naturopathic Healing Handbook

The Naturopathic Healing Handbook

Michael Schwartz

Inner Health Books

Naturopathic Healing Handbook
By Michael Schwartz

Published By
Inner Health Books
6003 Randolph Blvd
San Antonio, TX 78233

Editor: Mallory Clay
Page Design: Mallory Clay

**Publisher's Cataloging-in-Publication
(Provided by Quality Books, Inc.)**

Schwartz, Michael, 1943-
    The naturopathic healing handbook / by Michael
Schwartz.
    p. cm.
    Includes bibliographical references.
    ISBN 978-0-9796884-4-7

1. Naturopathy.   I. Title.

RZ440.S39 2012   615.5'35
                          QBI12-600008

Disclaimer

The information in this book is designed to help you understand and take care of yourself and others when necessary. It
is not intended to diagnose, treat or cure any condition. You
may want to consult with a healthcare practitioner and follow
their advice and guidance; though hopefully you are working
with a naturopathic or homeopathic physician. Ideally, you may
want to transition from pharmaceuticals or allopathic medicine
to homeopathic medicine, and then progress to naturopathic
support, which is in keeping with following the path of nature
and nurturing the body back to balance and homeostasis.

Table of Contents

Introduction

This book is an accumulation of information gathered over my years in the health food industry. I first became involved around 1975. I had the good fortune to be educated by the retailers I serviced and I have since learned many approaches to health and healing.

At the end of my consumer events, such as seminars or lectures, I am always asked if there is a book with all the information I talked about. Thanks to audience requests, I have assembled here some of my writings and included much of what I have learned and experienced along the way.

This book is filled with information that truly works—pure and simple. I have utilized this information for many, many years and have seen these nutrient combinations work on a personal level, as well as with family members. As a Mind/Body nutritional consultant, I had the opportunity to work with these concepts and nutrients, and from those experiences I created the supplement company, Michael's® Naturopathic Programs.

I know this information has ways to help you get back on the path of excellent health. Enjoy!

The Causes of Disease

In my understanding, a few key factors are the basic causes of disease. First and foremost is diet. The American diet is loaded with saturated fats, sugars, salt, and the biggest culprits – chemicals. Chemicals are applied in many different ways. The long and short of it is chemicals can and do corrupt the body as it is making new cells. The body will use whatever is in the bloodstream as building material.

If your bloodstream is laden with chemical structures that are alien to the body, and they become part of a process, they will alter your cells or the genes within and keep them from operating correctly. Once the DNA of the cell is corrupted or the genes malfunction, the stage is set for aging and disease, up to and including cancer.

Another group of causes are viruses. Viruses do not live outside of a host, but once inside a host, they burrow into a cell, alter the DNA, manipulate it, and make replications of themselves, to the point that the cell explodes and your body is then loaded with viruses. Some viruses can overwhelm the immune system. In time, with most viruses, the immune system will identify them and have a plan of action for eliminating them. This is one of the key reasons why it is so vital to have a healthy immune system.

Another cause of disease is the emotions. The emotions can create a lot of biochemical change in the body. Suppressed anger, resentment and/or frustration are examples of energies that have biochemical affects on the body. This is why, on some levels, it is good to vent so that negative feelings do not build and eat you up, creating ulcers or the like.

Stress too can create disease. Stress will compromise your vitamins and your minerals, especially calcium, which you need for many different transactions. One should keep the body slightly alkaline, because germs (as a catch-all) can thrive in an acidic environment. The American diet is comparatively acid rich. Proteins, such as meat, fish, fowl, nuts, grains and dairy leave an acid "ash" in your bloodstream. Calcium is vital in reducing the acidity, which is why it is essential to have minerals in your system to keep your body in a more alkaline state.

Another cause of disease is free radical damage. Free radical damage, or singlet oxygen as it has also been called, takes place when an atom is looking for an electron to balance its outer orbit. Sometimes, more specifically, it is the oxygen atom. In seeking an electron and stealing it from wherever it can, it creates an imbalance elsewhere. In turn, that may create other ramifications, such as cellular damage. This is one of the fundamental causes of aging. This is discussed in-depth in the Antioxidant section.

The Body's Structural Levels

The human body operates from several levels of structural organization. The broadest level is the body as an organism, with all parts of the body functioning together to make the organism work. The structure is then broken down into systems, such as the digestive system, which is comprised of several organs and functions that work together toward a common goal. Many organs, the next structural level, perform functions in more than one system. For instance, the pancreas is part of both the endocrine and the digestive systems.

Organs are composed of two or more types of tissues, the next level of structure. Cells are the basic structural and functional units of the organism. Among the many types of cells in the body are nerve cells, muscle cells, and, of course, blood cells. Each type of cell is unique in its construction. However, they each contain organelles, such as the nucleus or mitochondria, which perform specific functions geared toward the construction and operation of the cell.

The smallest level of structure in the body is the chemical level, which includes all the atoms and molecules essential for life. Carbon, hydrogen, oxygen, nitrogen, potassium, sodium and calcium are some examples of the types of atoms that create and maintain life on the chemical level. Atoms combine to form molecules, such as vitamins, fats, carbohydrates and proteins. These molecules, in turn, combine to form structures at the cellular level.

Almost every function within the cell involves a protein. There are thousands of different kinds of proteins and each performs a specific function, such as providing the structure of the cell or the capability of movement for the cell. Proteins are also important for their function in chemical reactions. Chemical reactions occur when chemical bonds are made or broken as atoms, ions or molecules collide with each other and change occurs within the cell. The chemical reaction cannot occur without the help of a specialized group of proteins, known as enzymes.

How to Protect the Body

Diet

The ideal diet would be 80 percent raw, 15 percent cooked and 5 percent junk. An easier approach is 60 percent raw, 30 percent cooked and 10 percent junk. Allowing for the junk takes away the resentment energy associated with deprivation.

Raw foods, fruits and veggies should be organically grown. Eat fresh sprouted organic seeds and whole grain products, such as millet and brown rice. If you are going to eat meat, make sure it is free range and grass fed. Grains are sprayed with chemicals and, therefore, those chemicals are in the animal eating them.

With fowl, you will want to eat more turkey than chicken. Chicken has more fat and that is where the toxins are stored. When it comes to seafood, refer back to Deuteronomy or Leviticus for dietary rules. Eat deep sea fish with scales. Seek to avoid fresh water and farm-raised fish, as these have a tendency to be more polluted. As for dairy, less is best. It causes phlegm and mucus in the intestinal tract and that will impede uptake of nutrients.

Water is an important nutrient, so drink plenty of it. Try to drink distilled or deep spring water, and add some fresh squeezed lemon juice.

Whenever possible, eliminate all fried, fatty and greasy foods and caffeine, sugar, salt and white flour. If you are a parent giving your child a chewy vitamin made with sugar or corn syrup, you are continuing the addiction to sweets. Look for stevia, zyltol or lo han as substitutes if you need a sweetener.

In addition to moving towards a vegetarian-style diet and minimizing the bad dietary items and habits, be sure to build your supplementation program with a strong high potency multiple vitamin, plus a strong mineral that you take in the evening -- your vitamins in the morning for energy throughout the workday, your minerals in the evening to calm and relax the body. You will sleep better as well.

Acid/Alkaline

A lot has been said and written about acidity and alkalinity. The bottom line is that your body is designed to be alkaline. You want your body to be more alkaline than acidic; the reason being that germs and cancer thrive in an acidic environment.

Proteins, nuts, grains and dairy deposit an acid residue in your bloodstream. The quickest way back to alkalinity is dried figs. However, a vegetarian-style diet is the ideal diet, because it will automatically make it easy for the body to maintain an alkaline state.

Fruits and veggies are fundamentally alkaline. The only vegetables you really want to be aware of are the nightshades: potatoes, tomatoes, bell peppers and eggplant. These are not good for people with gout and/or arthritis. The more fruits and veggies, the more alkaline the body, and the healthier you will be.

Antioxidents

Antioxidant compounds, in the form of vitamins, enzymes and elements, lessen the deterioration that free radicals inflict on our body's cellular machinery and genetic material. Some antioxidants are water-soluble while others are fat-soluble. Their solubility determines where they can travel and what reactive oxygen species they can quell.

Free radicals are electrically charged molecules that have an unpaired electron, leaving the molecule unstable and highly reactive. These incomplete molecules actively seek other molecules to bond with and "steal" an electron from, which, in turn, becomes unstable[1]. These radicals have an inherent ability to cause random, irreversible change in biological systems that can have very serious physiological results.

The billions of cells in the body are constantly exposed to these renegade radicals, which are created by normal body chemistry and other external sources, such as chemicals in the food, water, air pollution and cigarette smoke.

The damage inflicted on the body attributed to free radicals is believed to be wide-ranging and a major deterrent to good health. The body goes to great lengths to absorb essential elements necessary to keep a sufficient level of protection against the cell damage caused by oxygen-free radicals.

Antioxidant Functions and Factors

Antioxidants trap, deactivate and destroy free radicals, preventing the damage they can cause[2]. Antioxidants are, in effect, the body's kamikazes, called upon not only to function in their role as vitamins, but they are also pledged to neutralize themselves, if necessary, to win the battle of the cells.

Antioxidants, also called reducing agents, render radicals neutral in one of two ways. They can either react with and eliminate the radical or donate one of its own electrons to compensate the imbalance[3]. Either way, it is oxidized itself and, therefore, spent.

The group of compounds that function as antioxidants include well known vitamins such as vitamin A (beta carotene), C (ascorbic acid) and E (alpha-tocopherol). Other lesser known substances in our diets, such as selenium, manganese and superoxide dismutase, also function to inhibit free radical formation[4].

The antioxidant vitamins are interactive in that they work together to complement each other during situations of biological stress. Vitamin C, a powerful reducing agent itself, spares vitamin E and beta carotene until its own reserve is depleted[5]. Vitamin E and selenium appear to work synergistically in preventing oxidations[6]. The enzyme superoxide dismutase appears to be highly effective in removing superoxide radicals, including fatty acids, formed by several oxidation systems[7]. Although several vitamins are antioxidants, one cannot substitute for the other[8].

How the Body Protects Itself

Your body is under constant attack. Cells are being damaged because of all the chemicals in the air, water and food, not to mention microwave radiation. As the cells become damaged, mutations occur. One example is damaged DNA. When the cell divides, eachin half will be affected. The cells do not look right, nor do they know how to function properly.

Your immune system's phagocytes/macrophages work like the INS (Immigration and Naturalization Service). They check every cell to make sure it belongs in the body – it is self or non-self. Anything that is non-self, like the corrupted cells, do not belong in the body and the immune system will seek to eliminate it.

If there are too many corrupted cells, they overwhelm the immune system and cannot all be eliminated. Now you have "Murphy's Law" in effect, if something can go wrong, it will.

At this very moment you are manufacturing a million new cells. Eight hundred thousand are perfect. Two hundred thousand are corrupted. Your immune system was able to eliminate 150,000, now you have 50,000 cells that are corrupted and multiplying at different rates, depending upon the damage that has been done to the cell.

When I was in high school, there was a math problem of taking a penny and doubling the amount every day for a month. At the end of that time, you will have $5,368,709 and some change. Every cell creates two, two create four – you do the math and you will see that it is the same thing. You may not know you have a problem until you get to a billion cells because you have 50 trillion cells in your body.

Fortunately, the immune system has some help in its toiling. The lymphatic system contains several important structures and organs, as well as bone marrow, which is the site of lymphocyte (both T and B cell) production. Both the lymphatic and immune systems are involved in the body's war on foreign invaders. Since these systems are a complex interplay of many cell types and chemical functions, it is not surprising that poor nutrition can influence immune response.

Some of the essential nutrients and foods for proper immune system function include:

* **Vitamin A:** a fat-soluble nutrient which plays an important role in the immune system and the healthy formation of mucous membranes, a part of the body's outer protection against foreign toxins. The membranes release mucus in the linings of the mouth and nose, the digestive tube, and the breathing passages. Mucus is composed of water, cast off tissue cells, mucin, and white blood cells—the leukocytes. Leukocytes function as the catalyst for the B-cells and T-cells in the immune response process.

* **Pantothenic Acid:** serves as a part of the coenzyme A, which is essential for the production of energy, for the production of antibodies, and the healthy maintenance of the central nervous system.

* **Vitamin B-6:** is necessary for the maintenance of healthy skin, as well as the production of antibodies.

* **Vitamin C:** has many uses in the body. It is essential for the immune system, playing a role in the absorption of iron, and in the production of collagen.

* **Vitamin B-1:** plays a role in the nourishment of the immune system.

* **Vitamin B-2:** an important nutrient for the immune system because it aids in the formation of red blood cells and antibodies.

* **Vitamin E:** protects fat soluble vitamins and red blood cells. It is essential for the proper functioning of hair and the mucous membranes, both of which protect the body's openings.

* **Beta Carotene** is the preferred source of vitamin A because it is non-toxic, and ready to be converted to vitamin A only as the body needs it. Beta Carotene is one of the antioxidant nutrients, much like vitamin C, vitamin E and Selenium.

* **Zinc:** a component of zinc metalloenzymes, which are necessary for cell growth and the proper functioning of the immune system.

* **Folic Acid:** necessary for growth of all types of cells in the body, including white blood cells. It also takes part in the process of cell division and the healthy growth of glands, including the thymus.

* **Astragalus:** stimulates the immune system, macrophages, and the maturity of killer cells (phagocytes). Part of a historical Chinese formula[9].

* **Echinacea:** an herb that contains naturally-occurring small amounts of ascorbic acid, betaine, beta carotene, magnesium, niacin, selenium, zinc, polysaccarides, and flavanoids, all of which are important in the functioning of the immune system.

*   **L-Cysteine:** essential for the proper utilization of vitamin B-6 and serves as part of the body's heavy metal detoxification system.

*   **Rei-shi Mushroom:** stimulates the immune system, macrophages, and the maturity of killer cells (phagocytes). Part of a historical Chinese formula.

*   **Schizandra Berries**: stimulates the immune system, macrophages, and the maturity of killer cells (phagocytes). Part of a historical Chinese formula.

*   **Shiitake Mushroom:** stimulates the immune system, macrophages, and the maturity of killer cells (phagocytes). Part of a historical Chinese formula.

*   **Watercress:** stimulates the immune system, macrophages, and the maturity of killer cells (phagocytes). Part of a historical Chinese formula.

*   **L-Selenium**

*   **Inositol**

*   **Choline**

*   **Magnesium**

More on Diet

There is another biochemical transaction that the body performs when the diet is not of organic quality or is fed a chemical mixture of "food products." Additives such as artificial colors, flavors, flavor enhancers, preservatives, modifiers, and other chemical ingredients are added for various purposes.

These chemicals end up in the raw materials that cells use to create new cells, repair themselves and regenerate. Toxins have the potential to damage cells. The body is programmed to render the toxins harmless and eliminate them. Those that cannot be eliminated for one reason or another will be stored in fat cells and be incorporated into building material as the cells divide and create offspring, setting the stage for aging and disease or illness.

Here is a good approach to work with in cleansing and detoxifying your body: Cleanse your entire intestinal tract, blood and liver. Consider adding a fat metabolizer to enhance toxin elimination.

See the sections on Blood Toxicity, Liver, Digestion and Elimination, and Weight Loss.

How to Fix the Body

The following information will provide you with guidance on how to begin the repair process. Wherever there are imbalances, they can be corrected nutritionally through diet and supplementation in most instances. Obviously, when a physician or specialist is required they should be consulted.

Diet Recommendations

Very simple: Raw is best, as much fresh organically grown fruits and vegetables as is possible. As far as meat is concerned, it should be free range, organic grass fed because animal feed may be sprayed. Same thing with fowl; eat more turkey than chicken, as turkey has less fat. Fat is where toxins are stored. Reduce dairy intake, as it creates phlegm and mucous in the body.

Damage Control: Aging and Disease

Damaged and mutated proteins can cause cancer and inflammation. Protein molecules play a role in the appearance of skin, the ease with which joints function and artery function. Other important molecules attacked by oxygen-free radicals are enzymes, neurotransmitters, nucleic acids and phospholipids of plasma membranes[10]. Additionally, after disease or injury deprives a tissue of oxygen, the reintroduction of oxygen may cause further tissue damage due to the formation of oxygen-free radicals[11]. Free radicals and other reactive oxygen species are also formed at the sites of inflammation.

Free radical damage has played a role in a variety of degenerative conditions associated with aging[12]. The initiation of abnormal cell growth activated by oxidation results from chemical or physical damage to cellular genetic material (DNA) causing a mutation and growth of more such cells[13]. If a free radical were to bond with and borrow an electron from a DNA molecule, part of the body's very basic traits and information would be compromised. This would affect homeostasis, the balance and harmony within the body.

Nutritional Support

Antioxidants have been attributed to an abundance of biological abilities promising medical miracles. Some of this attention is desperately needed in order to gain respect among the medical profession regarding the role nutrition and vitamins can, and should, play in a person's overall health.

* **Vitamin C:** a powerful chemical antioxidant that helps promote the synthesis of collagen and conversion of iron[14]. In its role as an antioxidant, it both inhibits oxidative reactions and removes free radicals[15].

* **Vitamin A:** traps and removes reactive oxygen molecules and is a component of the body's primary defense against free radicals[16].

* **Vitamin E:** a fat soluble antioxidant that functions by interrupting free radical reactions[17].

* **Vitamin B-2:** participates in oxidation-reduction reactions in numerous metabolic pathways and in energy production via the respiratory chain.

* **Zinc:** a trace element that plays a role in the synthesis of DNA and RNA and in catabolism of RNA[18]. As with vitamin A, zinc functions in wound healing and plays a role in the body's ability to fight infection and destroy damaged cell.

* **Selenium:** a trace element of the metallo-enzyme that protects hemoglobin and some other body compounds from oxidative damage[19].

* **Rosemary:** has antioxidant powers.

* **Açai:** It has been shown that the antioxidants in **Açai** are able to enter cells in a useful form and that they can neutralize free radicals even at very low doses[20].

* **Pine Bark**

* **Resvertrol**

Naturopathic Approaches to Disease

Acid Reflux

Acid reflux, heartburn and indigestion are all pretty much the same problem. What is really happening?

When you think about it, what happens when you eat? Think about the size of your mouth for your body, and then think about the size of the mouth for each and every cell in your body. We call them receptor sites. You begin to realize that in order for a nutrient to get into the cell to help the cell feel good, or be healthy and function properly, the food you are going to give it has to be minute in size. So the question comes up, based on how well you chew your food, what is the size of the food when it hits your stomach? The next question is the size of the food. What size does it need to be when it goes into your intestinal tract? It is through your intestinal tract that the nutrient uptake occurs.

Here is what takes place. You eat a meal. Then your body goes into action. You may not feel this, but after you eat the muscles surrounding your stomach do two things. They squeeze the stomach to force the secretion of some digestive enzymes. They also agitate your stomach to enhance the disintegration, or breaking down, of the food to incredibly small particles for assimilation by the cells.

Your stomach is fundamentally a bag, and that bag can withstand the hydrochloric acid, where other parts of your body, such as your esophagus, cannot. It becomes irritated when it comes in contact with digestive acids. They could actually eat a hole through it.

Why is that some have heartburn and some do not? The answer is going to come down to minerals, because if you think about your stomach as a bag or a sac, and you think about the size of particles, then you realize that what has to take place in your stomach is that the food has to be broken down into pico-particles. They have to be infinitely small to be utilized by the cells, not to mention to enter the bloodstream through the intestinal tract walls. In order to do that, your stomach is shaken vigorously to mix all of the enzymes into the food to break them down into miniscule particles.

Your stomach has an opening at both ends and, when the agitation takes place, both ends are supposed to be securely closed. More often than not, the bottom sphincter is always closed, until it is time for nutrients and the chyme to migrate into your intestinal tract. However, the top valve (the top of the bag) should also close so that in the agitation process there is no blowback up into the esophagus. But, because of poor mineralization, the muscles are not getting the message they require, so they are not closing completely. Therefore, during the agitation process you are getting blowback and consequently you have acid reflux. So, multi-minerals are part of the answer.

There are a few health food companies that make products to alleviate the indigestion or the heartburn almost immediately. Some of the ingredients, like slippery elm and marshmallow, not only soothe the irritation or the esophagus, but will also help the healing of it. The truth of the matter is that the body is the healer, if you give the body what it requires. A quick liquid approach, which is also good for hiatal hernias, is aloe vera gel after meals.

Nutrients and Herbs for Acid Reflux

The following will assist the body in alleviating heartburn and speed healing of the esophagus:

* **Slippery Elm bark:** slippery elm bark is wonderful for removing mucus and phlegm from the intestinal tract. Also known for its soothing effect on membranes.

* **Marshmallow root:** known for its soothing effect on membranes.

* **Okra:** an old time favorite for acid and ulcers.

* **Complete multi-mineral**

Acne

Understanding the root causes of acne and eliminating the contributing factors is important to teens and adults. Doing so provides the necessary confidence to get a handle on life and turn negative situations around. If you catch it early enough, you will be able to positively influence the outcome and may be able to avoid the scarring that accompanies many cases of acne.

Acne is defined as a breakout of pimples, usually occurring in or near the oil glands of the face, neck, shoulders, or upper back. While the exact medical cause is unknown, certain bacterium do exacerbate the condition.

The first consideration in dealing with acne is to eliminate the contributing factors. What elements combine to create acne? Consider that old adage, "You are what you eat." The typical American diet centers on instant, prepackaged, frozen everything, fried foods, milk and cheeses, meat, and meat by-products —guaranteeing a large intake of saturated fatty acids. Saturated fatty acids are fats found mainly in beef, lamb, pork, veal, and whole milk products. Other sources are plant oils like cocoa butter, coconut oil, and palm oil. Margarine and hydrogenated shortenings also contain high amounts of saturated fatty acids. It is wise to avoid all products with hydrogenated oils.

When the body is laden with fats and other types of con-sumed toxins, it tries to remove them. This process involves the blood, lungs, kidneys, bowels and, of course, the skin. The blood carries the fats and toxins to every part of the body for elimination. The skin eliminates whatever it can via the drops of perspiration that ooze from the skin's pores. During times of stress and uncertainty, acne can become aggravated.

Skin

Perspiration consists of water with salt (sodium chloride), phos-phate, urea, ammonia and other waste products. These wastes, removed from the body's interior, can become food for the millions of microbes that live on the skin's surface. When the wastes are laden with impurities from the diet, the pores become clogged, microbes flourish, and acne can set in. Consequently, the pores must be kept clean and open. This means that the body must also have a clean diet and a regular supply of nutrients in order to manufacture healthy replacement cells for the skin.

Blood

In addition to supplying the body with life-sustaining nutrients, the bloodstream is also involved in waste removal. As old cells die or are destroyed by various natural processes within the body, they must be removed, along with organic waste that cells generate. If these wastes remain, problems can result, in-cluding acne and other types of skin eruptions. The skin is the body's largest organ of elimination, after all!

Liver

Liver cells seek to render harmless substances such as alcohol, nicotine, other toxins and various substances introduced into the bloodstream via the intestines. What cannot be rendered harmless is then stored in fat.

Dietary Changes

The logical starting point for cleaning the body's interiors and preventing most incoming toxins is the diet. Eat as many living, organic foods as possible: fresh fruits and vegetables, such as celery, garlic, carrots, and spinach; freshly sprouted seeds; and whole grain products like millet and brown rice. Eliminate all sugar, white flour, salt, caffeine, and fried, greasy, fatty foods from the diet.

Water is an important compound so drink plenty, preferably distilled or very deep spring water with some freshly squeezed organic lemon juice. This is good for the liver, helping to keep it clean from fatty deposits, plus it has alkalinizing effects.

Nutritional Support

Vitamins A, D, E, K and some of the B complex group are necessary in diets to maintain skin and hair health. The following information is provided to help you better understand the role that certain nutrients play in the overall health of the skin and the body.

Nutrients and Herbs for Acne and Skin Concerns

The following will assist the body in cleansing the blood, skin, and liver, and will speed healing of acne conditions:

* **Niacinamide:** A buffered form of niacin, this B-complex nutrient helps promote growth and repair. It participates in maintaining skin health by facilitating reactions that dilate the arteries and capillaries that carry blood to cells that construct skin. Cells are kept healthy by the blood being able to bring in fresh building material and carry away toxins.

* **Vitamin A:** Important for the skin and for maintenance of the outer layer of tissues and organs. Good for healthy hair and the growth and repair of body tissues. Used successfully in the treatment of acne[21].

* **Zinc:** Plays a fundamental role in normal tissue development, including cell division, protein synthesis and collagen formation[22].

* **Burdock Root:** An all-around blood purifier, strongly diuretic and diaphoretic. Cleanses the body of toxins; markedly enhances liver and gall-bile functions.

Allergies

An allergy is an exaggerated or abnormal reaction to something in the environment. Triggers can be substances, situations or physical states, In medical terms, these triggers are called allergens.

The allergens in foods are somewhat of a mystery to medical science. According to an article about them in Modern Nutrition in Health and Disease, it is largely unknown why some food proteins are more allergenic than others.

Allergies are labeled, identified, and classified by the degree to which and how the body's cells react to specific allergens. They are further divided based on how soon the body responds to the allergen, either a quick or a delayed response. An example of the delayed type of allergic reaction can be seen in contact with poison ivy. After being exposed, it normally takes a day or two for the rashes to appear.

Rashes are a common symptom of allergic reactions. Other symptoms include watery, swollen eyes, lung or nasal congestion, itching, fever, and even vomiting. For some people, the reactions can be fatal.

Allergy sufferers tend to have imbalances in their biochemistry, and in almost every instance, this can be traced back to an immune problem.

Symptoms manifest once the immune system fails to eradicate the allergen that has entered into the body. The immune system identifies everything that enters the body as either friend or foe. Allergies flourish when the immune system is not functioning at optimum levels. Even food allergies are believed to be an adverse reaction involving an immune response.

Nutrients, Herbs and Other Substances for Allergies

For support in eliminating common symptoms of allergies, including watery eyes, runny nose and sneezing, incorporate the following ingredients into your nutritional program:

* **Manganese:** Is involved in a wide variety of metabolic functions and helps certain white blood cells carry out the process of phagocytosis, the ingestion and destruction of toxins or other invaders.

* **Potassium:** Potassium is wonderful for stimulating the kidneys into eliminating toxins from the bloodstream. Also reduces inflammation that may accompany allergies.

* **MSM (Methylsulfonylmethane):** A source of sulfur. Excellent for the immune system.

* **Zinc:** Necessary for proper immune system function.

* **Vitamin A:** Essential for the immune system.

* **Vitamin B-6:** Reduces inflammation that may accompany allergies.

* **Vitamin C:** Stimulates immune response and is essential for the proper functioning of the immune system.

* **Pantothenic Acid:** This nutrient helps to nourish the adrenal glands; the stress centers of the body which are tied directly to the proper functioning of the immune system.

* **N-A-C (N-Acetyl-Cysteine):** For detoxification.

* **Dandelion Root:** Wonderful for the liver, which helps in the detoxification process. Most allergens are alien proteins that the body has not identified; the liver helps in protecting your body from these allergens.

* **Bee Pollen:** Often used by people with allergies, especially those with airborne allergies. Introducing small amounts of bee pollen into the body is equal to what a physician does by introducing a small amount of an allergen into the body so that it builds a tolerance and, thus, helps get the allergies under control.

* **Stinging Nettle Leaf:** Traditionally used by herbalists for hay fever and as an expectorant to help loosen a cough.

Alzheimer's Disease (See Memory Problems)

Anxiety

Here is another situation with multiple causes. Fundamentally, all of the causes for anxiety will lie within your subconscious mind, because anxiety, as stress, is the result of how you respond to what you see and hear. Most of us have no idea what is really going on in our subconscious mind; only of what we are consciously aware. Consequently, we are responding to stimuli throughout the day that could make us anxious. This is not to mention the tendency of people to live either in the past or in the future, with hardly anyone living in the present. Because of that, it does make one prone to uncertainty or regret -- you could be anxious about a past action and uncertain about a future endeavor. These would cause anxiety.

Whenever there is stress, it is going to do multiple things: affect the adrenal glands, in which case not only does your blood pressure go up because of the stress factor and the anxiety, but your immune system also begins to crash, along with your adrenals, so that its efficacy is no longer top notch. This is one of the reasons why people are prone to illness when they are stressed out and anxious. It is easier to catch a cold because your immune system has crashed with your adrenal glands.

The way around all this is a specific formula of pantothenic acid and Vitamin C. These are the two main nutrients that support your adrenal glands. Additionally, pantothenic acid is essential because it is the precursor to coenzyme A, which stimulates energy production in the mitochondria within the cell. Pantothenic acid is also essential if you are concerned with osteoporosis, because in one of its chemical pathways it becomes betaine hydrochloride. That is essential for allowing the calcium ion to be carried into, if you will, the bone matrix. Obviously, betaine hydrochloride is also a digestive enzyme. Additionally, pantothenic acid, through another chemical conversion, becomes pantethine, which is something that helps to emulsify cholesterol.

In addition to supporting the adrenals, make sure that multi-minerals are a part of your program. These are best taken in the evening, half an hour before retiring.

Take a high potency B complex. Stress will deplete your vitamins and compromise your minerals. If you take a B complex, you will know you have ample nutrition to help your body support itself in dealing with these issues.

Nutritional Support

Minerals play an important role in the transmission of impulses between the nerves and the muscles. Minerals are part of all body tissues and fluids. They are important factors in keeping physiological processes going. They act in nerve responses, muscle contractions, regulating electrolyte balance and the making of hormones.

The following information is provided to help you better understand the role that certain nutrients play in the overall health of the nerves and muscles of the body. These nutrients and foods are:

* **Calcium:** a mineral which is necessary for healthy, strong bones and teeth. Other functions of the calcium ion include its influence in neuromuscular excitability, cellular, and transmission of nerve impulses.

* **Magnesium:** essential for the normal metabolism of potassium and calcium.

* **Inositol:** necessary for hair growth, the metabolism of fats and cholesterol and for the formation of lecithin.

* **Niacinamide:** a B-complex nutrient that promotes growth and the proper functioning of the nervous system.

* **Vitamin B-6:** necessary for hair growth, the metabolism of fats and cholesterol and for the formation of lecithin.

* **Valerian Root:** great nervine. Excellent for calming and relaxing.

* **Skullcap:** great nervine. Excellent for calming and relaxing.

* **Hops:** great nervine. Excellent for calming and relaxing.

Arthritis

Arthritis has been called "everybody's disease" because it affects, directly or indirectly, almost everyone sooner or later. It is America's leading crippling disease, affecting one in seven people, or one in every three families. A million people develop arthritis each year[23]. Presently, about 30 million Americans are afflicted with this disease, of whom, three million are limited in their usual activities[24].

Rheumatoid Arthritis (RA)

Rheumatoid Arthritis (RA) is a systemic autoimmune disease that involves chronic inflammation and tissue destruction that begins in the synovial membrane of the joints. This type of arthritis is a widespread inflammation affecting both large and small joints. Rheumatoid arthritis is characterized by fatigue, pain, stiffness, deformity (which may be severe) and limited body functions. This disease is progressive. However, the symptoms may spontaneously disappear only to reappear again at a later time[25].

Osteoarthritis

Osteoarthritis, also known as deformant arthritis or degenerative joint disease, is the most common form of arthritis. It may follow injuries and other diseases of the joints and also could be influenced by congenital and mechanical derangements of the joints. There is degeneration of the articular (joint) cartilage, followed by sclerosis of the underlying bone, which triggers inflammation and pain in the surrounding joint. The early stage of the disease is marked by stiffness and can progress to a feeling of "soreness"[26]. There is usually minimal inflammation[27].

Osteoarthritis is chronic, however, it may become progressive in its course, limiting movement of affected joints; most often the hands[28]. It appears most frequently in older people and may develop from ordinary stresses or wear-and-tear on joints[22].

Nutrients Affected

Renewed interest in dietary factors in arthritis was generated by reports that some patients appear to have alleviated their symptoms by means of diet changes[30]. Ideally, you should eliminate the nightshade family of foods, such as eggplant, bell peppers, tomatoes and potatoes. Also, reduce amounts of protein, grains and nuts. The only nuts an arthritic can eat are almonds and cashews.

The disabilities and chronic diseases of these patients possibly interfere with their nutritional status, because of physical limitations and even depressed emotions[31]. Therefore, it is advisable to provide the nutritional supplementation necessary to maintain a state of homeostatic balance.

Most of the drugs used in treating rheumatic diseases have gastric toxicity. Abdominal pain is the most frequent manifestation, and nausea and vomiting may also develop and nutritional consequences can occur[32]. The following are some of the nutrients that may become compromised due to rheumatoid arthritis, osteoarthritis or the medications used to treat the symptoms thereof.

Essential Nutrients

*   **Vitamin C:** essential for the synthesis of collagen, the main extracellular protein of connective tissues. Numerous studies have shown low levels of ascorbic acid in the plasma and blood cells of people with RA. These are findings that have been confirmed by assays[33]. While the reason for the low levels has never been clarified, it is possible that therapy, particularly aspirin, may increase the rate of clearance of ascorbic acid, lowering the plasma levels secondarily[34].

*   **Vitamin E:** the most important lipid-soluble antioxidant, as it protects the integrity of normal cell membranes[35].

*   **Zinc:** People with RA have lower serum levels of zinc than normal individuals or those with other rheumatic diseases[36]. Gold salt therapy (any of several compounds of the metal gold used in the treatment of rheumatoid arthritis)[37] may decrease plasma levels of zinc. Low zinc levels have also been reported in patients receiving corticosteroid therapy[38].

*   **Vitamin B-6 (Pyridoxine):** Approximately 40 drugs (e.g. some oral antibiotics and penicillamine) are known to affect the metabolism or bioavailability of this water soluble vitamin[39].

* **L-Histidine**: This essential amino acid serves as a neuro-transmitter in the permeability process of blood capillaries, which allows for proper feeding of the joints' connective tissue[40]. The plasma of people with RA has lower levels of free sulfhydryl groups and decreased levels of histidine compared to normal individuals, whereas, levels of other amino acids remain in the same range as in normal subjects[41]. The decreased levels of histidine correlate with the degree of clinical activity of the RA, as measured by various parameters that affect the disease activity, such as the duration of morning stiffness, among other factors[42].

† **Vitamin D:** Since mineralization of the skeleton requires an adequate supply of vitamin D[43], supplementation of vitamin D is highly recommended for those with any kind of arthritis[44].

* **Calcium:** Is a mineral that plays a crucial role in metabolism, muscle activity, and nerve functions[45].

* **Magnesium:** A mineral needed to help consolidate and strengthen the bones, and is a vital component of all body cells, promoting many metabolic reactions and conversion of electrical potential in nerves and muscles as well[46].

* **Folic Acid (Folacin):** A water-soluble vitamin which aids in the breakdown and assimilation of protein, and assists the conversion of amino acids. Methotrexate - a chemotherapeutical agent – sometimes used as an NSAID to treat rheumatic diseases, is an antagonist of folic acid, causing massive shortages of this vitamin[47].

* **Vitamin B-12 (Cobalamin)**

Another NSAID used to treat RA, Sulfasalazine, inhibits the absorption of folate[48]. It has been suggested that those taking either drug be given folate each day[49].

Special Dietary Considerations

Eliminate tomatoes, eggplant, oranges, grapefruit, all white flour products, fried foods, meat, chicken (reduced if not omitted), preservatives and artificial colors/ flavors, sugar, salt.

Increase the consumption of raw vegetables: carrots, celery, parsley, cucumbers, garlic, alfalfa sprouts. Fresh fruits: bananas, peaches, pears, watermelon, plums, red grapes, cherries, papaya, pineapple. Whole grains: buckwheat, millet, soybeans.

Drink plenty of corn silk tea and/or alfalfa tea.

Asthma (See Congestion and Sinus Problems, Emphysema)

Backaches

Several factors contribute to backaches, such as stress, strain and injury. When there is stress, whether it is emotional or physical, it creates a nutritional demand upon the body. In most instances, the body is already at maximum output based on dietary intake. This often causes an imbalance, and muscle fatigue or cramping can be the result.

Another set of causes can be strictly nutritional. In this case, it is a matter of inadequate amounts of minerals and B-complex vitamins, both of which are essential because of their roles in electrical message conduction.

Nutrients for Backaches

Here are the nutrients that ease backaches and help the muscles return to balance and harmony:

*   **B-Complex Vitamins:** Essential for proper nerve function and communication; they participate in the communication necessary for the muscles to relax as well as to contract.

*   **Calcium:** Mineral that help the electricity of communication flow between the nerve endings and the receptor

sites on the cells. This allows the cells to get the message of how to perform, facilitating all of the cells working in harmony, in this case to relax the back muscles.

* **Magnesium:** see Calcium

* **Potassium:** see Calcium

* **Proteolytic enzymes:** are ideal for reducing all inflammation of the back muscles as well as inflammation anywhere in the body.

Halitosis (Bad Breath)

Bad breath can be caused by many different things. Poor dental hygiene obviously is one. Poor digestion is another, because food may be rotting in the stomach. When that system is open at the top, then that aroma can be emitted when you breathe, when you exhale, when you communicate. There could also be gum disease. With this in mind, a good mouth wash would be something centering on goldenseal root, pau d'arco bark, black walnut hulls and myrrh resin -- all of which will kill bacteria. Oregon grape root has the same efficacy as goldenseal root. Using a mouth wash on a consistent basis is the ideal.

Since I am focusing a little on the mouth, cracks at the corners indicate a need for vitamin B2. I would take 100 mgs twice a day.

Baldness

There are three basic causes of baldness: One is poor circulation to the scalp. Another possible cause is that the arteries are clogged to some degree and there is not enough blood getting to the hair follicles in the scalp. Therefore, they starve to death and hair growth is lost. (See the section on High Cholesterol.)

Another cause of baldness is stress. The stress can be physical or emotional because that, too, affects the muscles. This is where the body tightens the muscles curtailing the amount of blood flow to the scalp. In this situation minerals would also be advisable to take as additional support for dealing with the stress. (See Stress and Tension. Also, Nerve and Muscle Function.)

Allergies are another cause. This is when the immune system identifies the hair follicles as non-self, as aliens, and seeks to destroy them, eventually resulting in baldness.

In an allergic situation, or an allergy-related baldness, and auto-immune baldness a.k.a alopecia, I do not think that the hair follicles can be re-stimulated to grow hair. If it is a matter of poor circulation, then massage the scalp while shampooing your hair; certainly cholesterol metabolizing nutrients (see High Cholesterol section), as well as stress-relaxing nutrients (minerals), will be of assistance.

Bladder Issues

Normally when there is a bladder issue it is an infection. Generally, the rule of thumb is to drink lots of cranberry juice. One of the things cranberry does is prevents the bacteria from adhering to the urethra wall. I would also ingest lots of Vitamin A, Vitamin C, and zinc as a way of killing the infection, as well.

Some of the essential nutrients for proper functioning of the immune system include:

*   **Vitamin C:** has many uses in the body. It is essential for the immune system, playing a role in the absorption of iron, and in the production of collagen.

*   **Vitamin A:** a fat-soluble nutrient which plays an important role in the immune system and for the healthy formation of mucous membranes, part of the body's outer protection against foreign toxins. Beta Carotene is the preferred source of vitamin A because it is non-toxic and is converted to vitamin A only as the body needs it. Beta Carotene

is one of the antioxidant nutrients, much like vitamin C, vitamin E and Selenium.

* **Echinacea:** an herb that contains naturally-occurring small amounts of ascorbic acid, betaine, beta carotene, magnesium, niacin, selenium, zinc, polysaccharides, and flavanoids, all of which are important in the functioning of the immune system.

* **Wood Betony Craig**

* **Wild Lettuce Leaf**

* **Garlic**

* **Bioflavonoids**

Blood Toxicity

Blood is the life stream of the body, affecting every cell and system. The bloodstream is a conglomeration of different elements, each working in a specific way to keep us alive. The blood system is composed of plasma, a sticky substance made up of 95 percent water and 5 percent nutrients, proteins, hormones, and waste products, among other components.

The cleansing process of the blood is carried out by the body's detoxification system. Without such a system, the body would become toxic and unable to support itself.

Four examples of the body's detoxification systems are the respiratory, defecatory, perspiration and urinary systems. The respiratory system expels wastes in the form of carbon dioxide, which is exhaled from the lungs. Solid organic wastes and dead blood cells are expunged by the defecatory system, and the remaining waste products, transported by plasma, are expelled by the urinary system and sweat.

Nutrients are the substances needed by the body's tissues to sustain their normal function and growth. The principal nutrients are sugars, fats, amino acids, vitamins and minerals. All these are dissolved within the plasma and transported to each cell within the body.

The primary proteins in the plasma serve either as part of the clotting mechanism, as part of the immune system, or as transporters for nutrients or hormones. Hormones are chemicals used to regulate many of the body's functions. They are produced in the endocrine glands and then released into the bloodstream to their various target organs elsewhere in the body.

Nutritional Support

For the complex operation of the body, the blood requires a constant source of nutrients. Nutrients are essential for the feeding of tissues of the body and are necessary to sustain its intricate functions as it constantly reproduces new cells. Each cell requires nutrients for their formation and specific function and when each cell within the body functions properly, homeostasis is achieved.

Some examples of essential foods and nutrients in the blood's/body's cleansing process are:

* **Zinc:** considered a trace element because the body requires only small amounts to function. Though the body requires only small amounts of zinc, inadequate levels can affect proper detoxification. One of these important enzymes, carbonic anhydrase, of which zinc is an integral part, acts as a carbon dioxide carrier, especially in red blood cells, and catalyzes the reaction[50].

* **Manganese:** necessary for the function of glutathione synthetase, an enzyme needed for the body to make the detox conjugator glutathione from glycine[51]. Glutathione functions in various redox reactions: (1) in the destruction of peroxides and free radicals, (2) as a cofactor for enzymes, and (3) in the detoxification of harmful compounds.

* **Iron:** essential in its role in the transportation of oxygen in the body and permits cellular respiration to occur[52].

* **Molybdenum:** Certain molybdenum metallo-enzymes oxide and detoxify various compounds that play a role in uric acid metabolism and sulfate toxicity.

* **Echinacea:** Significantly stimulates the body's own blood-cleaning system. It destroys the germs of infection directly and bolsters the body's defenses by magnifying the white blood cell count. This herb is also good for lymphatic cleansing.

* **Red Clover:** An herb that acts as a wonderful blood detoxifier/purifier.

* **Burdock Root:** An all-around blood purifier, strongly diuretic and diaphoretic.

* **Gotu Kola:** A blood purifier, glandular tonic, and diuretic as well as an oxygen carrier.

* **Yellow Dock:** Primarily affects liver function and the health of related organs, increasing their ability to strain and purify the blood. In addition, the herb has antibacterial properties.

Special Dietary Considerations

Eliminate as much of the preservatives, food colorings and additives as possible. Avoid tap water and meats that are not well prepared or cooked.

Increase celery, onions, garlic, carrots, parsley and as much raw vegetables and fresh fruit as possible.

Drink clean distilled water throughout the day. Chaparral tea or any of the herbs in this formula that can be found as a tea.

Bruising

Some people can just walk by a desk, barely touch it, and the next thing you know they have a black and blue mark. Whenever there is bruising, this is an indication that the capillaries are very fragile. What strengthens your capillaries are the bioflavonoids, rutin and hesperetin, part of the C family of nutrients. If you are easily bruised, the ideal supplement is a super C complex; in other words, 1000 mg of Vitamin C, 500mg of bioflavonoids, with rutin and hesperetin. That will take care of any bruising.

Bursitis

The suffix "itis" simply indicates that inflammation is present. Whether it is bursitis, arthritis, diverticulitis or any other "it is," it indicates inflammation.

One of the best ways to resolve inflammation in the body is through the use of proteolytic enzymes. These enzymes have the ability to "see" a mutated protein, which is one of the fundamental causes of inflammation. Proteins are generally formed with a chain of amino acids. However, when an improper amino is part of the chain and it folds, that is when you have a mutated protein, which creates inflammation. In fact, it is known that mutated proteins are one of the root causes of cancer.

In this instance, the ideal proteolytic enzymes are those that are enteric coated so they will dissolve in the intestinal tract, which is an alkaline environment, versus dissolving in the stomach and being utilized like a digestive enzyme. Enzymes that dissolve in the stomach, which is an acid environment, will be utilized in the digestion of food. You want to have the enzymes dissolve in the intestinal tract so they can migrate into the bloodstream and hunt down mutated proteins. They do this by reading the chain of aminos, seeing the particular amino that does not belong in that chain and excising it, allowing the aminos to fold into a proper protein, thereby eliminating inflammation.

Cancer

Besides AIDS, cancer is one of the most devastating diseases plaguing mankind today, claiming millions of lives each year. The most frightening thing is that the numbers are growing, and cancer is getting progressively worse. In some medical reports cancer is now the number one cause of death for people under the age of 85.

Medical science tells us that researchers have absolutely no idea what causes this disease. From a physiological perspective, it can be seen that cancer is mutated or uncontrolled cellular growth. So, the medical community does know what causes cancer however is reluctant to admit it. This reluctance is based on economic and political considerations.

Doctors who say that cancer can be cured through dietary changes and increased nutritional supplementation are drummed out of the medical community. To cure cancer or to admit its cause would create financial havoc in the world economy because we would not be able to change quickly enough to a non-cancer-causing system of economics. Everything we are currently doing would become invalid. Therefore, the truth of the situation is played down, rebutted, and ignored, and the people who bring up the truth are generally disgraced or eliminated.

The truth is easy to see when you examine the facts of cancer. There really is no mystery.

Cancer is a general term for forms of new tissues that have no controlled growth patterns. These tissues, at a cellular level, are due to a growth of mutated cells. Mutated cells are generated within the body when certain cells are affected by mutagens. Mutagens are any chemical or physical agents that cause a gene change (mutation) or speed up the rate of mutation.

Chemicals are identified as a major source of mutagens. What are all of the sources of these chemicals? Unfortunately, chemicals are everywhere—in our food, the water we drink, the air we breathe and the substances we rub on our skin. It is virtually impossible to eliminate them from our world at this stage. In fact, the number and amount of chemicals in use is so staggering that we may have created a cancerous situation for the earth as well, which—if we do not correct our ways quickly—will kill the planet. Earth is a living entity, too, and can only take so much abuse and neglect.

In addition to polluting the planet, we have disrupted its own natural feeding and replenishing cycle. We have depleted the soil of nutrients and contaminated it, so that it no longer supports life in the same abundance it once did. The vegetables, grains, and fruit produced using these soils are nutritionally depleted, as are the animals that graze on the grass growing in it. All living things that require the soils as a source of nutrients are undernourished because the soil is sick, and so are we.

Why doesn't the government regulate the harmful chemicals and ban them from human consumption? As for government involvement, or the lack thereof, could it be that commerce in the pursuit of profits and dollars is more important than the conservation of life—the planet's and ours?

Cancer is…

In essence, cancer is a disease born out of many different factors including man-made chemicals. They create a distrubance at a cellular level. The chemicals enter the body through the food chain as well as the air we breathe and the drinks we consume. In an internal atmosphere, a chemical "fire" is ignited. As it burns and smolders, the "smoke" or cells of it spread, and as it spreads it consumes or infects everything in its path. Eventually, if left unchecked, the "fire" will destroy the body.

Cancer does not require oxygen to thrive and grow; an illness of this type is called an anaerobic infection. The opposite of an aerobic organism or process that thrives only in oxygen, an anaerobe is a microorganism that can live without oxygen.

In seeking to understand the symbolic implications of cancer, just as we did with arthritis, we need to go back to definitions of cancer contained in medical textbooks and references, such as The Merck Manual, where we get the perception that the cause of cancer is "unknown." When something is unknown in life, it is usually because it is not understood. With that concept in mind, new questions arise: From what frame of reference have we historically looked at this condition? What guidelines and points of reference did we use? Did we ask all the right questions?

Let us look at how a disease grows within the body. What causes a healthy body to move to a state of ill health? The answer is simple; it is a result of something the person brings into the body. There are four primary avenues of introduction: food, water, air, and light.

The abundance or lack of each of these elements leaves its own distinctive mark on health. For example, the fluorescent lighting to which most of us are exposed daily during our working lives has cumulative, detrimental effects. Over time, the skin becomes yellow and heavily creased.

Where natural sunlight is concerned, there are two distinct outcomes. Some people have health problems because they do not get enough natural sunlight. On the other hand, we are told that too much exposure to the sun increases skin cancers. Maybe it is not the sun at all, bur rather the pollution in our air and food. Maybe the pollutants in these substances, once in our bodies, are reacting with the sunlight and creating a chemical reaction we call cancer. (For more insights regarding sunlight, see Arthritis.)

Every day, you and I breathe air and drink water that contains some type of chemical pollutant. At any given time, we are eating, drinking, or breathing minute pieces of toxic pollution that alter the systems within the body, and create conditions that cause weakness or vulnerability, compromising the integrity of certain systems and leading to many health problems, including cancer.

By the time an individual is seventy years old, he or she may have had a form of cancer up to six times. One difference between those who manifest it and those who do not is the immune system, your body's first line of defense.

If you understand symbology, you are constantly aware and in prime defensive mode. Even though there is not a defensive attitude, you know that you need to be in control. You know everything you are dealing with and can make the proper decisions, because you see it clearly and deal with it from a position of strength. This leaves no room for failure, which can lead to feelings of guilt, resentment, or possibly even blame, and this continual barrage of strong emotions contributes to the development of cancer.

Warning signs for cancer may be found in altered in bowel or bladder habits, non-healing sores, unusual bleeding or discharge, thickening or lumps in the breast or elsewhere, indigestion or difficulty in swallowing, an obvious change in a wart or mole, a nagging cough or continuing hoarseness.

The First Step

The first step in physically dealing with cancer is to modify your diet. Look at the foods that you eat on a daily basis, and if yours is the typical American diet, the need for dietary change is obvious. Begin immediately to increase your regular intake of fresh, organically grown raw vegetables and fruits.

Fresh foods are full of energies that are better at promoting vitality than cooked, frozen, or canned foods. Organic farming methods also mean that fewer chemicals will ultimately be introduced into the body. Cooked foods, on the other hand, produce a lifeless type of energy in the body. Heat destroys the vitamins and enzymes within foods that make life happen within the body.

Let us go back to the concept of "unknown" causes again. We can begin to see that the substances, foods, and pollutants that enter the body play a role in affecting our health; our diet plays the major role.

If you knew that certain foods were bad for you, would you continue to eat them? For most people, the answer would be an immediate and resounding no. However, some people will continue to eat the foods they know may be detrimental to their health. Why? The answer lies in the human thinking process, wherein can be found the true cause of cancer as well as other diseases. Every action and reaction that you have begins within your mind and there is not one interaction that you can think of that is not directly related to a particular thought.

Every choice you make, including your food selection, is the result of emotional associations and desires buried deep within your subconscious mind. Advertising messages use this psychological tendency to their advantage in crafting their commercial messages.

New Theories

In some medical circles, cancer is being examined as a viral disease that flourishes due to the body's lowered defenses. This is brought on by an improperly functioning immune system and stress. As research continues to focus on this aspect of the disease, it is becoming very clear that stress is a major factor in disarming the body's immune system.

Stress taxes the adrenal glands, which secrete hormones that carry messages to the other glands on how to perform or what to manufacture. When the adrenal glands are stressed and begin to falter, the immune system also falters. All the body's glands are tied together in a complex system, and each and every aspect of life within the body is interdependent. This is why it is so important to maintain a proper nutritional balance. In this way, you are providing the system with the ingredients it requires to function properly in a state of optimum health, thus eliminating opportunities for disease to take hold.

Nutrients, Amino Acids and Herbs to Support the Immune System

Suffice it to say that every nutrient is absolutely essential in the battle against cancer. There are some that are especially important, such as selenium, astragals and the Chinese mushrooms: Reishi, Shiitake, Maitake and Cordyseps. All of these are wonderful for strengthening the immune system, and that is one of the things you must do with cancer.

The best nutritional approach to prevent or combat cancer is a comprehensive, daily, foundational program that includes all nutrients available today. To strengthen immune response and increase adrenal stamina, include the following nutrients, amino acids and herbs:

*   **Vitamin A:** Should always be included in any formula designed to fight disease/infections. Nothing is more stimulating and nourishing for the thymus gland than vitamin A, which affects cell-mediated immunity. Vitamin A and beta-carotene have been found to protect against cancer in humans. Higher intakes of beta-carotene[53] and vitamin A[54] are associated with a lower risk of cancer, and beta-carotene has been found to have specific anti-tumor activity in animal studies[55]. Synthetic forms of vitamin A have been used to correct pre-cancerous conditions[56] and to treat cancer itself[57].

* **Folic Acid:** necessary for growth of all types of cells in the body, including white blood cells. It also takes part in the process of cell division and the healthy growth of glands, including the thymus.

* **Pantothenic Acid:** nourishes the adrenal glands, which, in a weakened state, can allow the immune system to become lowered. It is also involved in energy production.

* **Vitamin B-6:** vital because of the role it plays in antibody and red blood cell production. The presence of vitamin B-6 also increases the number of T-cells. T-cells are phagocytes, white blood cells that are matured by the thymus gla

* **Vitamin C:** should always be included in any formula designed to fight disease/infections. Vitamin C, or ascorbic acid, has its own history when it comes to fighting disease and infections. It has prophylactic and therapeutic effects in pathologic conditions. Studies indicate vitamin C modulates cyclic nucleotide levels in B-cells and T-cells, a process that may mediate immune reactions.

* **Selenium:** a trace element of the metallo-enzyme that protects hemoglobin and some other body compounds from oxidative damage. It helps to preserve tissue elasticity. The availability of selenium in foods depends on several factors, including the level in soil where crops are grown.

* **Zinc:** plays an important role in nourishing the thymus gland as well as liberating vitamin A from the liver. Zinc deficiency impairs phagocyte function, cellular immunity, humeral immunity, and their inter-communication.

* **L-Cysteine:** an amino acid active in the production of antibodies

* **Echinacea:** a very powerful immune booster that stimulates interferon production and helps to cleanse the lym-

phatic system thoroughly. Echinacea normalizes the white blood cell count and stimulates intracellular processes that destroy pathogens such as viruses and bacteria[58].

* **Astragalus, Ligustrum, Reishi Mushroom, Codonopis:** chosen because of their particular power and influence on the immune system. These Chinese herbs play a major role in the development of white blood cells. They literally engulf and digest bacteria that are too big for antibodies.

Candida Albicans (Yeast Infection)

Candida albicans is a yeast fungus that occurs naturally in the body in small quantities. However, when this organism has the chance to grow and proliferate, a yeast infection can erupt. This often happens when there is a deficiency of our "good" bacteria allowing for overgrowth of other bacteria and yeast. Antibiotics are often the culprit in allowing for this condition.

Antibiotics kill the friendly flora in the intestinal tract, creating a vacuum of sorts, and since Candida is the first to grow back into the intestinal tract, it will dominate there because of its own natural ability to multiply.

Additionally, there is an opportunity for Candida and toxins to enter the bloodstream via a condition called "leaky gut." As a result of malnutrition and the ingestion of harmful substances, cells within the intestinal lining die, creating holes through which these materials can pass.

Candida does not perform the same supportive function for the body as do the friendly bacteria, such as acidophilus, and it can actually drain the body of energy. As a by-product of metabolism, friendly bacterium produce B-vitamins for the body, while Candida does not.

B-complex vitamins are involved as co-enzymes in energy production as well as other enzymatic processes within the body, they help the body to develop and maintain energy, as well as function properly. When the body and the intestinal tract are overwhelmed by Candida, an inadequate amount of B-vitamins is produced, causing the body to go into somewhat of a dive, both on a physical and an emotional level.

Consequently, the person who has Candida throughout the intestines and bloodstream has a hard time generating and maintaining strength and energy. In order for the body to free itself of this infestation and rebalance, it must become nutritionally fit. This means establishing both a strong immune system and a hostile environment for the yeast. Creating a hostile environment means depriving the yeast colony of its food sources and attacking them full force with natural substances that will destroy them, and also means strengthening and stimulating the immune system to "clean house."

Nutrients, Amino Acids and Herbs to Eliminate Yeast and Bacteria

The following will boost your body's immune system and increase elimination of toxins, yeast, and bacteria:

* **Vitamin A:** Nourishes the thymus gland, increasing its size and antibody production.

* **Vitamins B-1, B-2, and B-6:** Involved in nourishing the adrenal glands. When the body is sick or under attack, it places stress on the adrenals, which can, in turn, stress and deplete the immune system. By keeping the adrenals well nourished, it should help to prevent illness or hasten recovery time.

* **Pantothenic Acid:** Nourishes the adrenal glands, which helps to support the immune system.

* **Zinc:** Essential for natural antibody production.

* **Black Walnut:** contains natural properties that kill fungus and bacteria.

* **Buckthorn Bark:** Helps in cleansing the system of toxic and waste material.

* **Corn Silk:** Helps in cleansing the system of toxic and waste material.

* **Dandelion Root:** Improves liver function. Bile and certain enzymes produced in the liver aid in maintaining proper intestinal flora.

* **Echinacea:** Cleanses lymph system and improves antibody production.

* **Garlic:** A wonderful anti-bacterial, anti-fungal, anti-microbial agent and is great for killing Candida.

* **Goldenseal Root:** contains natural properties that kill fungus and bacteria.

* **Myrrh:** contains natural properties that kill fungus and bacteria.

* **Pau D'Arco:** contains natural properties that kill fungus and bacteria.

* **Uva Ursi:** Helps in cleansing the system of toxic and waste material.

* **Cascara Sagrada:** Helps in cleansing the system of toxic and waste material.

* **L-Cysteine:** Involved in natural antibody production.

Yeast Control Diet:

Foods You Can Eat

All Fresh Vegetables	Greens	All Fresh Fruits	Meat and Eggs*
Asparagus	Kale	Apple	Beef
Beets	Spinach	Avocado	(limited)
Broccoli	Mustard	Banana	Chicken
Brussels Sprouts	Collard	Grapes	Turkey
Cabbage	Turnip	Pear	Lamb
Carrots	**Nuts & Seeds**	Pineapple	Veal
Cauliflower	Brazil Nuts	Apricot	Egg
Celery	Almond	Berries	Tuna
Corn	Brazil Nuts	Cherries	Oysters
Cucumbers	Cashews	Mango	Salmon
Eggplant	Filberts	Necatrine	Clams
Green Peppers	Pecans	Plum	Squirrel
Onions		Orange	Rabbit
Parsley	**Whole Grains**	Papaya	Quail
Tomatoes, Fresh	Corn		
Peas, Beans, Le-	Millet	**Oils (cold pressed)**	Duck
gumes	Barley		Goose
Squash, Zucchini,	Oats	Almond	Cornish Hen
Acorn & Butternut	Cereal Grains &	Apricot	Pheasant &
Squash	Muffins(containing	Almond	other game
White Potatoes	no yeast, honey or	Avocado	birds
Sweet Potatoes	sugar)	Corn	
Parsnip		Linseed	
Radishes		Olive	
Okra		Safflower	
Parsnip		Sesame	
		Sunflower	
		Butter	

* Except bacon, sausage, ham, hot dogs or luncheon meats.

Yeast Control Diet:

Foods You Cannot Eat:

* Sugar and sugar-containing foods: sucrose, fructose, mulattoes, lactose glycogen, glucose, mannitol, sorbitol, galactose, monosaccharide and polysaccharide. Also avoid honey, molasses, maple syrup, date sugar and turbinado sugar.

* Yeast, breads and pastries.

* Alcoholic beverages: wine, beer, whiskey, brandy, gin, rum, vodka, etc. Also abstain from fermented beverages, such as cider and root beer.

* Malt products.

* Condiments, sauces and vinegar-containing foods: mustard, ketchup, Worcestershire, Accent, etc. Also horseradish, mince meat, tamari and sauerkraut.

* Processed and smoked meats.

* Dried and candied fruits.

* Leftovers: mold often grows on leftover foods that are refrigerated. Freezing is best.

* Fruit juices.

* Coffee and tea: includes herb teas.

* Melons.

* Edible Fungi: all types of mushrooms.

* Cheeses: also buttermilk, sour cream and sour milk.

* Yeast: Brewer's yeast and baker's yeast.

* Vitamins and mineral that contain yeast.

* Nuts: Peanuts and pistachios usually contain mold.

Canker Sores

Canker sores are ulcers that form on the inside of the mouth. When you get one of these, it is an indication that your bloodstream is too acidic. The acidity is the result of digestion of protein foods, such as meat, fish, and fowl; also occasionally from nuts, grains and dairy.

In terms of nuts and acidity, the only nuts that someone with gout or arthritis could eat, or should eat (if they are going to eat nuts), are almonds and cashews.

One of the best ways to deal with canker sores is to immediately buy a bag of dried figs. Figs are one of the most alkalizing foods known. Next up would be umeboshi plums, which is a macrobiotic food. Drink lemon water, it is good for alkalizing and it is also wonderful for stimulating the liver and helping it to work more efficiently and correctly. Also, you could take a Vitamin A pearl, puncture it, and place the oil inside your mouth over the canker sore (every day application), until heal the sore heals.

Cataracts

Three-fifths of all people between the ages of sixty-five and seventy-four show the beginning signs of cataracts, and by age eighty, they cloud nearly everyone's vision to some degree.

Removing and replacing eye lenses damaged by cataracts is the most common surgery in the U.S., with some 650,000 of the procedures performed annually at a whopping cost of one billion dollars! Some experts contend that if preventive measures could be taken to delay cataract formation by an average of ten years, then the number of operations could be cut in half.

Various types of stressors can result in cataracts. Besides the aging process itself, illnesses like diabetes are one cause. Frequent exposure to X-rays, microwaves, the intense heat from blast furnaces or welding torches, and the sun's ultraviolet rays are among other known causes.

Protein and vitamin deficiencies can be a contributing factor as well as drugs, such as cortisone, or even a severe blow to the eye. More common causes suggested by the Journal of the American Dietetic Association[59] are insufficient levels of water and other fluids in the body, and the excessive consumption of milk in later adulthood.

A study published in the New England Journal of Medicine[60] reports minerals and vitamins can prevent diabetic cataracts. Chief among those recommended are calcium and magnesium, plus all vitamins from the B-complex group. Additionally, vitamin A is very important in preventing the eyes from drying out[61]. At least one study also reports that the sulfur amino acid glutathione likewise protects against cataracts[62].

There is yet another natural approach to eliminating cataracts. One of the older European approaches is to place eight to ten drops of raw, unfiltered, uncooked honey in the eyes at bedtime. The honey's enzymes will eat away at the cataract. In the morning, one simply washes the eye with warm water.

Nutrients, Amino Acids and Herbs for Eye and Vision Support

The following will assist the body create healthy eye lenses, improve eyesight, and protect against damage caused by free radicals:

* **Vitamin A:** Vital to the formation of rich blood and maintenance of good eyesight. Essential in the formation of visual purple, a substance in the eye necessary for proper night vision.

* **Vitamin B-1:** Essential for proper nerve function.

* **Vitamin B-2:** Cataracts can easily be produced in laboratory animals by depriving them of this vitamin, also called riboflavin. A diet low in protein has also been linked to this

eye disorder. Riboflavin deficiency can also cause visual fatigue, a "sandy" feeling of the eyes, and inability to endure bright lights.

* **Vitamin B-3:** Used in many enzymatic reactions used to promote energy and blood flow.

* **Folic Acid:** Essential for cell division, and is necessary for healthy eye cells.

* **Inositol:** Helps to support healthy eye membranes.

* **Vitamin C:** Protects thiamine (B-1), riboflavin (B-2), folic acid, pantothenic acid (B-5), and vitamins A and E against oxidation.

* **Bioflavonoids:** Contain citrin, hesperidin, rutin, flavones, and flavonals. Essential for the proper absorption and use of vitamin C.

* **Vitamin E:** An antioxidant that protects against the damaging effects of many environmental poisons present in air, water and food.

* **Calcium:** Needed for nerve and muscle action.

* **Magnesium:** Activates more enzymes in the body than any other mineral.

* **Selenium:** A component part of glutathione peroxidase, a free radical scavenger, which protects the eye from damage. Pre-radical damage to the eyes is often related to the formation of cataracts.

* **Zinc:** The vascular coating of the eye contains more zinc than any other part of the body.

* **Chickweed:** Useful for eye infections (glaucoma, cataracts), hemorrhoids, blood diseases (leukemia, tetanus), and eczema.

* **Eyebright:** Useful for sore, inflamed eyes in which there is considerable stinging and irritation associated with watery-to-thick discharges, or conjunctivitis (pink eye).

* **Red Raspberry Leaves:** Astringent for the eyes (reduces mucus in them); also reduces hyperglycemia (excess glucose levels in the blood), which may be linked to cataract development.

* **L-Arginine:** Amino acid that are basically free radical scavengers. Hunts free radicals and nurture the eye lens.

* **L-Cysteine:** Amino acid that are basically free radical scavengers. Hunts free radicals and nurture the eye lens.

* **L-Glutamine:** Amino acid that are basically free radical scavengers. Hunts free radicals and nurture the eye lens.

* **L-Glutachione:** Protects metabolism in the eye's lens by preserving the physicochemical equilibrium of its proteins, maintains the molecular integrity of the lens fiber membranes, and protects membranes and organelles from oxidation.

* **Niacin**

* **Pantothenic Acid**

* **Vitamin B-6**

* **Vitamin B-12**

* **Vitamin D**

* **Ginger**

Charley Horses

Charley Horses are basically muscular cramping. Look at the section on Cramping, or go straight to Minerals.

Most of the time when you have cramping, palpitations, spasms, it is caused by a lack of minerals in the diet and in your supplements. This is one of the reasons I constantly stress high potency nutrients. The low doses will not provide enough sustenance to bring balance and harmony to the system.

Chronic Fatigue

I am of the belief that chronic fatigue, hypoglycemia, and fibromyalgia are all interrelated. I feel that because hypoglycemia is so often misdiagnosed and not dealt with from a proper point of nutrition, it ends up elevating itself or escalating into chronic fatigue. Also, whenever there is hypoglycemia, there will almost always be Candida. In this case, you are talking about an infestation in the intestinal tract. Candida crowds out, and may even diminish, your probiotics (your friendly bacteria) which manufacture your B vitamins. With no probiotics in your intestinal tract, you are not going to be able to manufacture B Vitamins. Your vitamins are integral for energy production within the body. So, you can see the onset of the chronic fatigue.

One of the key ingredients against chronic fatigue will be pantothenic acid. Also, strengthening the adrenal glands will help. One thing that must be understood is that nothing stands alone. When you look for a magic bullet in one product that you think is going to do everything for you, it is an illusion, and you set yourself up for disappointment in a situation like that. Nurse your adrenals, high B vitamins and lots of pantothenic acid.

Nutritional support for chronic fatigue

* **Pantothenic Acid:** Acid plays a role in the release of energy from carbohydrates; in gluconeogenesis; in the synthesis and degradation of fatty acids; and in the synthesis of such vital compounds as sterols and steroid hormones and porphyrins[63].

* **Folic Acid:** a water-soluble B vitamin that is important in both the production and synthesis of nucleic acids (RNA

and DNA). Because the daily folate requirement is hinged to the daily metabolic and cell turnover rates, its need is increased by anything that increases the rate of either, such as physical stress. Although folates are readily present in nearly all natural foods, it is highly susceptible to oxidative destruction and 50 to 95% of the folate content of food may be destroyed by cooking or other processing[64]. Folic acid's metabolic role is interdependent with B-12 and both are required for cell growth and reproduction in the body[65].

*   **Vitamin B-12:** a water-soluble vitamin necessary for the synthesis of nucleic acids (RNA and DNA), the maintenance of myelin in the nervous system, and the proper functioning of folic acid[66]. Two important relationships exist between B-12 and folic acid. First, both are required for growth, which is dependent on cell replication, and cell replication is dependent on DNA synthesis. Vitamin B-12 is also necessary for the transport and storage of folate in cells[67].

*   **Vitamin C:** occurs in large concentrations in both parts of the adrenal gland[68]. It is essential in the production of the two active hormones, epinephrine and norepinephrine, by the adrenal medulla. Even though the adrenals are rich in vitamin C, upon secretion of corticosteroids large amounts of vitamin C are lost from them[69].

*   **Siberian Ginseng:** is an adaptogen; meaning it makes everything work better.

*   **Ashwagandha Root:** for energy.

*   **Juniper Berries:** for the pancreas and insulin production.

*   **Licorice Root:** or the adrenal glands and stress.

*   **Curcuma longa**

Circulation Problems

The circulatory system is the lifeline of the body, carrying oxygen and food (vitamins, minerals, fats, proteins, and carbohydrates) that our body requires for health and performance. A well-fed body is healthy and vibrant. This system also facilitates the removal of toxins from the body.

Keeping these lifelines (the arteries) open and free-flowing ensures that all the glands, organs, muscles, nerves, brain and skin remain well fed. Problems arise when the arteries begin to clog, reducing the amount of blood available for all functions and structures.

Clogging results from excess fats or cholesterol in the bloodstream, which can clump together to form ever-larger fatty deposits. As they grow in size, these deposits capture minute particles of minerals (ions) floating in the bloodstream. This is the beginning of the conditions that can manifest in arteriosclerosis, commonly called "hardening of the arteries," where excess fatty deposits cling to the arterial walls. Ion after ion, the passages are narrowed.

To avoid major circulatory problems and the possible heart disease associated with them, it is important to identify the most common symptoms of poor circulation. They include:

* Hair loss

* Memory loss

* Hearing loss

* Cold hands and feet

* Numbness in fingers and toes

* Arms and legs that "fall asleep" easily

If three or more of these symptoms are present, it is time to take action to get those arteries open to their maximum dimensions once again.

The first step should be to reduce the intake of those foods that contribute to excess fats or cholesterol in your blood, such as refined carbohydrates and hard fats, such as hydrogenated, transfats, and saturated. Remember, the fat/cholesterols is the "cement" that binds the minerals in your blood to the arterial walls. Cholesterol also has the positive function of cementing up or "patching" weak spots in the vessels, this is where the "cementing" begins. Cholesterol is used for cellular integrity, hormones and natural vitamin D to mention a few uses.

The second step would be to start a nutritional program that will dissolve existing excess fat/cholesterol deposits, which should improve blood flow to the heart and head, which will help provide more oxygen to your brain and forestall dementia or worse, and extremities.

Nutrients, Amino Acids, Herbs and Digestive Enzymes for Circulatory Support

The following will assist the body in opening arteries, dissolving cholesterol and triglycerides, reducing water content, re-assimilating calcium from arterial walls, regulating cholesterol, equalizing blood pressure and toning the heart.

* **Vitamin B-6:** As a natural diuretic, it reduces water and water pressure from the cardiovascular system and is excellent at metabolizing fats, proteins, and carbohydrates.

* **Choline:** Lipotropic nutrients that work as "fat burners," dissolving excess fat and cholesterol.

* **Inositol:** Lipotropic nutrients that work as "fat burners," dissolving excess fat and cholesterol.

* **Vitamin D:** Essential for calcium assimilation. Most people with poor circulation are also calcium-starved, resulting in part from calcium becoming lodged in the cholesterol plaque in the arteries.

* **Vitamin F:** This nutrient is also known as unsaturated fatty acid. It is essential for dissolving cholesterol and saturated fats in the bloodstream.

* **Niacin/Niacinamide:** Excellent for opening up arteries to provide more blood and oxygen to the heart, head, and extremities.

* **Magnesium:** A mineral that supports calcium assimilation.

* **Apple Pectin:** Helps to regulate cholesterol and also draws toxic metals out of the blood. It is said that apple pectin contains electromagnetic properties.

* **Capsicum:** Stimulates circulation and purify the bloodstream, increasing blood flow and regulating blood pressure.

* **Garlic:** Stimulates circulation and purify the bloodstream, increasing blood flow and regulating blood pressure.

* **Ginger:** Stimulates circulation and purify the bloodstream, increasing blood flow and regulating blood pressure.

* **Hawthorne Berry:** Valuable for its heart-strengthening properties.

* **L-Methionine:** An amino acid that acts as a "fat burner." Essential in the production of lecithin.

* **Betaine HCL:** A digestive aide that supports calcium assimilation.

* **Pantothenic Acid**

Colds and Flu

Do you know anyone who has never had a cold, the flu, or some kind of respiratory infection? A cold is a contagious viral or bacterial infection that affects predominately the upper respiratory tract, and has specific symptoms such as a stuffy nose, watery eyes, low fever, and an overall achy feeling, usually in the joints.

While the flu also has specific symptoms, unlike a cold, the flu can attack either the respiratory or intestinal tracts, and either a viral or bacterial infection can spread, circulating in the bloodstream to any area in the body. Both colds and the flu generally spark mucus congestion in the lungs or sinus cavities.

In every infectious situation, whether it is a cold or flu, there is usually a fever. This can also be generated by nerve disease or cancer. The basic metabolism of the body increases as antibodies are formed and they create an army of fighters to combat the invading force of bacteria, viruses or other toxins. This is when the body creates a fever, also called hyperpyrexia. If a fever is left to run its course without being controlled, in extreme cases it can cause convulsions. Dangerously high fevers are seen in the most serious and contagious diseases, particularly in young children and older adults.

Nutrient and Herbs to Assist the Body in Fighting Colds and Flu

The following will assist the body in expediting immune response for colds or infections:

* **Vitamin A (Beta carotene):** Preferred source of vitamin A because it is non-toxic and is converted to vitamin A only as the body needs it. Vitamin A is important in the maintenance of epithelial and mucosal surfaces and secretions as a form of primary defense. It is also important for healthy function of the thymus gland as well as other body systems.

* **Vitamin C:** Stimulates immune response and has a generally positive effect on the common cold.

* **Zinc:** Plays a fundamental role in normal tissue development, including cell division, protein synthesis, and collagen formation. This is very important in the production of antibodies.

* **Echinacea:** has natural antibiotic properties.

* **Garlic:** has natural antibiotic properties.

* **Goldenseal Root:** has natural antibiotic properties.

* **Comfrey Root, Fenugreek, and Slippery Elm Bark:** These three herbs are highly effective in breaking up mucus and phlegm in the sinus cavities and lungs. They are the perfect herbal complement to infection-fighting nutrients. In addition to its efficacy against mucus, slippery elm bark also has astringent and anti-inflammatory properties.

Congestion and Sinus Problems

Asthma and Emphysema

While congestion, asthma, and emphysema share some basic symptoms, these conditions also have individual traits that necessitate separate discussion. Let us begin by defining some terms. Congestion is an abnormal collection of fluid in the body, generally found in an organ. When we speak of congestion, we usually are referring to the type that makes breathing difficult, mainly mucus accumulation in the lungs. Sinus cavities can also become congested.

Asthma is a lung disorder marked by attacks of breathing difficulty, wheezing, and coughing, and causes thick mucus to be produced in the lungs. Asthma attacks can be triggered by stimuli such as allergens, infections, vigorous exercise, or emotional stress.

Emphysema is a lung disease categorized as a defect of the lungs. It causes over-inflation of the lungs and destructive changes of the air pouches which make the lungs become too rigid. When emphysema occurs early in life, it is believed that it is the result of an inherited defect or caused by damage to the air pouches.

Physical and mental symptoms associated with emphysema include anxiety, high levels of carbon dioxide in the blood, insomnia, confusion, weakness, appetite loss, congestive heart failure, fluid in the lungs, and lung failure.

Because the breathing difficulties experienced by persons with asthma can also cause undue stress on the lungs' air pouches, it seems logical that gaining control of asthma early in life is not only important for the immediate relief of symptoms, there may also be long-term ramifications relevant to emphysema. Since compromised air pouches figure prominently in the development of emphysema, by controlling or eliminating asthma early on it may be possible to avoid the full impact of emphysema as well.

Nutrients and Herbs to Support Immune Function and Breathing

To strengthen overall immune response and support the body in combating the symptoms associated with breathing congestion, include the following nutrients and herbs:

* **Vitamin A (Beta-carotene):** Due to its non-toxic nature, it is the preferred source of vitamin A, which is important in the maintenance of epithelial and mucosal surfaces and secretions as a form of primary defense. Beta-carotene is converted to vitamin A only as the body needs it.

* **Vitamin B-1, B-2, B-6, and Pantothenic Acid:** Involved in nourishing the adrenal glands. These nutrients play a vital role because of the strain illness or stress places on the adrenals. When the adrenal glands are taxed and depleted, the result can be an under-performing immune system that can lead to prolonged recovery times for any illness or condition attacking the body.

* **Vitamin C:** Stimulates immune response. It also has a generally positive effect on the common cold, fights bacterial

infections, and reduces the effects of some allergy-producing substances.

* **Folic Acid:** Has a direct nourishing and fortifying effect on the "front line" of the body's defense system.

* **Magnesium:** Helps regulate the body's acid/alkaline balance. The body becomes more susceptible to disease when the blood is acidic.

* **Zinc:** Plays a fundamental role in normal tissue development, including cell division, protein synthesis, and collagen formation. Zinc is very important in the production of antibodies, and plays an important role in nourishing the thymus gland, the "seat" of the immune system, and in liberating from the liver another source of thymus nourishment, vitamin A.

* **Slippery Elm Bark:** Both an astringent and anti-inflammatory, which helps to reduce inflammation in the lungs. It also works at removing mucus from the body.

* **Fenugreek:** A powerful herb used to support removal of mucus from the body.

* **Mullein:** Highly effective in breaking up mucus and phlegm in the sinus cavities and lungs.

* **Vitamin D**

* **Niacin/Niacinamide**

* **Potassium**

Constipation

Although constipation has many causes, diet is the major contributing factor. Certain medications are also known to be a causative factor for constipation. It is astonishing to look through the Physician's Desk Reference (PDR) and see how different drugs have side effects that can cause constipation.

One potential and often ignored cause is a compromised level of minerals. Another would be an obstruction somewhere in the intestinal tract, a condition so serious it would require a medical procedure to remedy.

The fundamental cause is the American eating habits and food manufacturing processes that have combined to render diets lacking in fiber, another major cause of constipation. People eat flesh food and too much processed food, especially bread, pastries, white rice and cereals. Most food products derived from grain do not incorporate the grain's protective fiber shell, which is often removed for better processing and quicker cooking.

Fiber has at least three important roles within the intestinal environment. Cellulose fiber breaks down and becomes foodstuff for some of the beneficial microbes that live within the intestinal tract. Fiber also acts as a gentle "broom" of sorts, sweeping against the intestinal villi, the fingerlike threads through which nutrients are absorbed into the bloodstream, and also moves matter along the digestive pathway to help ensure that nothing clogs the lining of the intestines.

Fiber in the intestinal tract acts as a triggering device. It absorbs water, swells, and pushes matter against the colon walls, which signals the brain to evacuate. Nerve endings within the intestinal wall sense the pressure and tell the brain to create the muscular motions that are necessary to move fecal matter through the colon. It is in this respect that a mineral deficiency can contribute to constipation. Minerals are essential for muscular contractions, so if minerals are low, the muscles will not efficiently move matter through the colon.

What some health professionals overlook is that many transactions within the body, outside of manufacturing and mitosis, are muscle-driven. Manufacturing refers to the glands' production of the enzymes and hormonal messengers that regulate and command the systems within the body.

Although we do not often think of it as such, constipation can be life threatening. As fecal matter sits in the colon, toxins from it are reabsorbed into the body. Constipation can be eliminated by increasing fiber in the diet, eating more organically grown raw fruits and vegetables, increasing liquid consumption—particularly distilled water and organic fruit and vegetable juices—and avoiding milk and soda.

Try not to consume liquids at meals, which dilute the digestive juices and could cause fermentation of foodstuffs, resulting in gas and bloating. Taking probiotics helps digestion, assimilation, and elimination.

Taking multi-minerals is also of primary importance because minerals participate in enzyme transactions as well as muscular transactions. Drinking aloe vera juice after each meal is another suggestion because this can act as a lubricant.

Do not eat onions from open salad bars, as they draw bacteria to themselves.

Finally, do not forget to include minerals in your supplement support and do your exercises, which benefits circulation to the entire body, including the muscles involved in digestion and evacuation.

Nutrients, Foods and Herbs for Constipation

*   **Calcium and Magnesium:** Both support contractibility and relaxation of muscle. This facilitates the muscular transactions necessary to move matter through the intestinal tract. They are also vital for proper elimination, as this too is controlled by muscles.

*   **Apple Pectin:** Along with other fibers, pectin is excellent for the intestinal tract. Fiber is beneficial for many different reasons, such as pushing matter along, absorbing toxins, and helping to absorb bile acids, which prevent the breakdown of fats and the absorption of water to help matter flow easily.

* **Butternut Root Bark, Prunes, Senna:** These herbs are well known for aiding in bowel movements. They act like laxatives without the addictive nature of those types of products.

Cramps

Cramps can occur in any muscle within the body. They are perhaps most often associated with menstruation in women or as a result of strenuous physical activity. Cramps happen when a muscle contracts but does not relax. What causes it to contract, and what prevents it from relaxing? The quick answer is minerals. Cramping can be caused by a lack of minerals, particularly calcium, magnesium, potassium, or phosphorus.

Calcium and magnesium, especially, are vitally important in muscular function because they are catalysts, acting like light switches to facilitate the flow of electrical current, and this electricity stems from thought. Minerals allow the electricity of thought to make the leap from nerve ending to receptor sites on the cells of the muscles, and they transport the electrical impulses that tell the muscle what to do—thought energy, if you will—so that the muscle will contract or relax accordingly.

Nutrients and Herbs to Support the Body in Dealing with Muscle Cramps

* **Calcium:** A mineral involved in neuromuscular excitability and transmission of nerve impulses. When calcium levels become low in the blood, increased neuromuscular irritability, seizures, and cardiac cramps are possible.

* **Magnesium:** Deficiency symptoms include muscle fasciculation (involuntary twitching), tremors, and muscle spasms to name a few.

* **Hops, Skullcap, Valerian Root, and Wild Lettuce:** All have calming, relaxing properties.

* **Phosphorus:** Essential for calcium assimilation.

* **Potassium:** Required to stimulate nerve endings for muscle contractions.

* **Vitamin D:** Must be present for the assimilation and utilization of calcium. Vitamin D is so effective in helping the body to assimilate calcium that it has been used by itself to dissolve joint and spinal calcium deposits.

* **Inositol:**

* **Niacinamide**

* **Vitamin B-6**

* **L-Tyrosine**

* **Passion Flower**

Diabetes

Diabetes is a metabolic disease affecting how the body uses glucose, or blood sugar. One indication of diabetes is that the person suffers from the constant need to drink fluids, but displays no other symptoms. An unconscious person with diabetes insipidus, or Type I, during surgery or accidental injury, will still produce great amounts of urine, so if enough fluids are not given, the patient becomes severely dehydrated and develops electrolyte and mineral imbalance.

Another type of diabetes is Type II diabetes mellitus. The disease tends to run in families, but may be triggered by outside factors such as physical stress, obesity and ingestion of too many refined carbohydrates.

The pancreas releases insulin when it is signaled by the adrenal glands when they detect a rise in sugar in the blood stream. Insulin also promotes the transport and entry of sugar into the muscle cells and other tissues while lowering the amount of sugar in the blood stream. When the pancreas does not produce enough insulin, the symptoms of diabetes mellitus develop, including weight loss, tiredness and lethargy.

As with diabetes insipidus, the symptoms in diabetes mellitus also include frequent urination and increased thirst, however these are often accompanied by weight loss and increased appetite. Sugar levels in the blood and urine will be high. In addition, the eyes, kidneys, nervous system, and skin may be affected. Infections are common and hardening of the arteries often develops.

There are several diabetes-linked complications, many involving the eyes or vision. For instance, diabetic amaurosis is a form of blindness that can be caused by bleeding into the retina. Cataracts are another vision problem that seems to be common in both Type I and Type II diabetes. Problems arising from poor circulation and infections are also a concern for those with diabetes. A related skin disorder, xanthoma, which produces yellow bumps on the skin in uncontrolled diabetes mellitus, disappears when the disease is brought under control.

When diabetes is present, the body cannot process all of the starches and refined sugars coming into the system from our diets. The pancreas, which has the sole responsibility of producing insulin for the body becomes overloaded. The emotional/mental aspects need to be changed, and this change is equal or even greater than the need to change the diet.

Nutrients, Foods and Herbs to Support Circulation and Insulin Production

The following will assist your body in increasing metabolism, insulin production, circulation to the extremities, and beta-cells in the pancreas; in opening arteries; and in neutralizing acidity in the blood.

* **Vitamin B-1:** Needed for carbohydrate metabolism.

* **Niacin/Niacinamide:** Aids in the metabolism of fats, carbohydrates, and proteins.

* **Chromium:** The primary role of chromium is to maintain normal levels of blood sugar (glucose) that act as fuel for the body. If glucose levels are high, supplementation lowers them; if levels are low, supplementation raises them.

* **Iodine:** A component of the thyroid hormone helps regulate the body's production of energy, promotes growth and development, and stimulates metabolism. Metabolism is a strong factor in the body's ability to burn fuel (glucose, fat).

* **Zinc:** Needed for the synthesis of insulin. Zinc binds to insulin and enhances its activity.

* **L-Glutamine:** An amino acid that lessens the craving for sweets.

* **Cedar Berries:** Used to stimulate the pancreas. If there are beta-cells left in the pancreas, where insulin is produced, the combination of herbs will stimulate them.

* **Goldenseal Root:** Supports lowering blood sugar levels.

* **Kelp:** Provides iodine, which is essential for thyroid hormone production. The hormones regulate metabolism helping to burn off some of the stored fat (energy). That is what fat is, stored energy, and too much of it becomes a problem.

Diarrhea

Diarrhea is a problem for both young and old. Regardless of the cause, when diarrhea is present, any food that has been ingested is rapidly expelled from the system. If it continues to the point of dehydrating the body, more than nutrients will be lost and the condition can become life threatening.

Stopping diarrhea as quickly as possible is of paramount importance. The best way to accomplish this task is by tackling the problem head-on. Since diarrhea is more of a symptom than a disease, we need to attack it symptomatically. The first step is to eliminate the parasite or germ causing the condition.

Next, increase the amount of fiber foods. You could also mix carob powder in food or drinks. This will gel the bowels and cause the stool to become firmer.

By stopping the diarrhea process, all food that is consumed will remain in the body longer, affording the system an opportunity to extract the nutrients it needs for replenishing.

In Mexico, where this condition is more common, the people do two interesting things. They squeeze fresh lemon juice over all salads before they eat them, and when diarrhea does strike, they eat plenty of cheese, which gels the bowels. Generally, what creates diarrhea is a bacteria or fungus within the intestinal tract that the body is trying to expel as rapidly as it can because the body's own intelligence has identified it as a threat to the body. With diarrhea, there is such a rapid expulsion of the liquid portion of the waste in the intestines that electrolytes are lost and nutrients are not absorbed into the bloodstream. It is also possible that the lack of nutrient uptake could be created by faulty digestion.

When you lose electrolytes and minerals, you set the body up for other problems because minerals are involved in enzymatic processes. Minerals are co-factors that allow biochemical processes and exchanges to take place, and are also catalysts that facilitate other transactions. When there is a mineral deficiency, the body will utilize what is available for the most essential functions. This can be problematic because the secondary and tertiary issues are not well cared for because there are not enough nutrients available to meet all of the nutritional requirements of the body.

Here is a chain of events that demonstrates what a lack of nutrients due to diarrhea can cause. Due to rapid expulsion, calcium uptake is diminished. Of course, this could also be the result of poor nutrition, where the pancreas and stomach lining did not produce enough digestive enzymes, then digestion would be impeded and nutrient availability is therefore limited.

The first signs of calcium deficiency are muscle aches, spasms and palpitations. This could manifest in many different ways, including a fatal heart attack.

Calcium is a conductor of electricity and chemical processes essential for life. When the electrical flow of the body is affected, health is compromised, and compromised health could be fatal. Another telltale sign is the slow process of clotting when you cut yourself.

When there is a lack of sufficient calcium ions in the bloodstream the body intelligence will pull calcium from the bones. This is done to try and keep the body in an alkaline state, and germs cannot live in an alkaline environment.

In addition, the process of supplying the bloodstream with calcium can cause osteoporosis. This is especially true if calcium supplementation is not used.

In dealing with diarrhea, two of the best things to do immediately are to consume carob powder and cheese. Carob gels the bowels, and cheese will literally gum up the system, slowing the loss of fluids and electrolytes.

Herbs to Support the Body in Combating Diarrhea

The following act as congealers and liquid-absorbing agents, helpful in solidifying the stool and regulating bowel movements following diarrhea:

* **Acacia and Carob:** Absorb discharges and soothes irritated linings of the intestines.

* **Bayberry, Blackberry, Rhubarb and White Oak:** All are known as powerful astringent herbs traditionally used by healers in combating diarrhea.

* **Charcoal:** Absorbs liquid and excess gas.

* **Garlic and Pau D'Arco:** Used to kill bacteria.

* **Cinnamon**

Dementia (See Memory Problems)

Depression

Depression is a difficult condition to understand. It often carries with it only the lone symptom of hypoglycemia (low blood sugar).

Taking only that into consideration (because there are so many different causes as to why a person could be depressed), hypoglycemia can be fixed by nourishing the adrenal glands. So, working on that, let's see if we can turn the situation around.

Nourishing and strengthening the adrenals is essential because there may be a lot of stress in a person's life. Because of the amount of stress, everything is overwhelming, and because it is overwhelming, one does not feel that they have the wherewithal to deal with it, which can lead to depression.

This could also lead to eating lots of sweets, giving oneself a reward, which would overtax both the adrenals and the pancreas, which would give a high energy effect from the sugar and then the crash – the insulin crash. This is when the depression would be at its worst and anger could also be present. The best way to fix this is by addressing the adrenals.

Nutritional Support

The following information is provided to help you better understand the role that certain nutrients play in the body's energy production. Those nutrients and herbs are:

*   **Pantothenic Acid:** serves as part of the coenzyme A, which is essential for the production of energy, for the production of antibodies, and the healthy maintenance of the central nervous system.

*   **Folic Acid:** necessary for growth of all types of cells in the body, including white blood cells. It also takes part in the

process of cell division and the healthy growth of glands, including the thymus.

* **Vitamin B-12:** helps form normal red blood cells and a healthy nervous system. It helps the body metabolize fats, carbohydrates and proteins.

* **Aspartic acid:** an amino acid used by athletes for endurance. A very small amount goes a long way.

* **Gotu kola:** a wonderful oxygen carrier, which is why it is also in memory nutrients. Your body utilizes oxygen as part of the energy consuming process and gotu kola is excellent for providing that.

* **Licorice Root:** goes straight to the adrenal glands, so it helps support the adrenal glands while it is dealing with the stress. This is optimal, because when the adrenal glands falter, so does the immune system.

* **Rhodiola:** has been used for hundreds of years in Siberia and Russia. It is excellent at regulating blood sugar levels.

Digestion, Assimilation, Utilization, and Elimination Issues

Good health is the result of many factors — the way we think, the air we breathe, the water we drink and the food we eat.

Two of these factors are summed up in the expressions: "You are what you eat," and "You are what you think." The types of food you eat determine the nutritional health of your body. If the food is predominantly cooked, then its nutritional value would be much lower than that provided by raw vegetables. If the diet lacks the fiber found in living foods and is heavy in dairy products or fats, such as hydrogenated oils or saturated fatty acids, you can bet that there will be difficulties, especially in regard to the food digestion, assimilation, and utilization process. These difficulties will be experienced across the entire channel of digestion, which is more like a canal or long tube with an opening at both ends. It includes the mouth, esophagus, stomach, intestinal tract, and colon.

Digestion

Digestion begins in the mouth. When you see, smell, or taste something, messages are transmitted to the brain, which signals the first step in the process: production and release of enzymes to aid in the digestive process by the salivary glands. As masticated or chewed food continues down the esophagus into the stomach, the second and most major enzymatic process takes place: the pancreas and stomach lining both secrete enzymes that ensure further digestion. The pancreatic gland produces enzymes that digest proteins, fats and carbohydrates.

The hormone insulin for the facilitation of sugar into the cells is also manufactured here. When problems arise in the pancreas, digestion is disrupted and constipation can result.

Once the enzymatic contributions of the stomach lining and the pancreas have been added, the resulting liquid, called chyme, moves into the duodenum for further digestion. When the chyme enters into the intestinal tract, the process of assimilation begins. At this point, the nutrients in chyme are molecular in size.

Assimilation

Complete assimilation depends on the small intestine being clean and having a thriving colony of friendly bacteria (a.k.a probiotics). Complete, effective assimilation depends on two factors. First is the quality of the food ingested: was it fresh, organically grown raw food, or did it come out of the freezer or a can? The second factor is the quality, or thoroughness, of the digestive process itself: to what degree has the food been broken down, and is the quality of the chyme such that the nutrients will be able to pass through the intestinal wall?

The amount of nutrients coming into the system and the amount assimilated determines your level of health, because everything you have assimilated into your bloodstream through the villi will now feed your individual cells. This underscores the need both for consuming good food and having efficient cleansing processes. Often, it is necessary to reinforce and supplement the natural cleansing process because of all the toxins entering the body. It creates a load over and above the normal wastes that the body produces in the feeding of the cells and removing the waste that they generate.

When the diet is not of organic quality or is overly processed, the body is being fed a chemical mixture of "food products" that is heavy in artificial colors, flavors, flavor enhancers, preservatives, modifiers and other chemical ingredients added for various purposes. These chemicals end up in the raw materials that cells use to repair themselves and regenerate, and many are toxins with the potential to damage the body. The body is programmed to render them harmless, eliminate them or store them in fat cells.

Toxins may first be broken down into harmless substances. What cannot be broken down and eliminated will be stored in the fat cells. What cannot be eliminated or stored will end up being incorporated into building material as the cells divide and create offspring, and this sets the stage for possible disease or illness.

Utilization

When we talk about utilization, we are talking about the availability of the nutrients in the bloodstream. Once nutrients are in the bloodstream, other issues and questions come into play, such as: Are there other nutrients that complement each other and that are vital and necessary for the utilization of other nutrients?

Much like nature, nothing stands alone. This is one of the reasons why "magic bullets" do not work. They block the symptom and never deal with the root cause of the problem. Utilization is about being able to utilize the nutrients within the body, not just assimilate them into the bloodstream. They can only be utilized by finding their counterparts, their allies and comrades, if you will, that work in conjunction with them.

Elimination

The body's overall elimination process involves four systems. The respiratory system is used for eliminating carbon dioxide, spent air, and other detrimental gaseous substances. The urination process is the result of the kidneys filtering liquid wastes out of the bloodstream. The skin uses perspiration to vent steam and liquids. Lastly, the intestinal tract passes all used and unused solid material from the body through defecation, completing the elimination process.

The solids, water, and gases are taken from the bloodstream, converted in the liver and then dispersed. The water and gases are placed back into the bloodstream for elimination, and the solids are passed through with bile into the intestinal tract for elimination.

The need to keep the intestinal tract clean and healthy cannot be emphasized strongly enough. Fiber plays an essential role in cleaning the intestinal tract, and this is why a diet rich in fiber is important. It can be supplemented with fiber tablets and powder.

Another vital aspect of cleansing is to eliminate any unnecessary mucus in the system. Mucus is created from dairy-based products, as well as some whole grains, and mucus can accumulate in the intestinal tract, blocking assimilation pathways.

Taking probiotics is one step you can take to ensure better assimilation. Probiotics are beneficial microbes that protect the host from foreign entities entering the bloodstream.

Additionally, they provide the body with B-complex vitamins, which help prevent disease. The best-known probiotic is lactobacillus acidophilus, which is found in yogurt, acidophilus milk and supplements. While probiotics could, and should, be consumed periodically to ensure a healthy bacterial colony, it is particularly important to take them after a course of antibiotics, which destroy friendly bacteria in the intestinal tract, allowing other forms to flourish. (See also Candida Albicans)

A clean colon aids proper elimination and helps to ensure there is no retention of toxic materials.

Nutrients, Enzymes, and Herbs to Support Digestion, Assimilation, Utilization and Elimination

The following supports the body in eliminating indigestion and heartburn, improving digestion, bettering intestinal health, eliminating mucus, and normalizing eliminations:

For the Pancreas:

* **Manganese:** Supports detoxification pathways. Stores of it are found chiefly in the human liver, kidney, pancreas, lungs, prostate gland, adrenals and brain.

* **Selenium:** Good for the liver and pancreas. It is a natural antioxidant and appears to preserve elasticity of tissue by delaying oxidation of polyunsaturated fatty acids.

* **Zinc:** Plays a part in the manufacturing of insulin in the pancreas.

* **Cedar Berries:** Stimulate the pancreas.

* **Dandelion Root:** Stimulates bile production, benefits the spleen and improves the health of the pancreas.

* **Gentian Root:** Its focus of activity is on those glands and organs involved in digestion, such as the liver and pancreas. It also works on the gallbladder.

* **Goldenseal Root:** Lowers blood sugar; stimulates the pancreas.

* **Licorice Root:** Strengthens the pancreas and spleen.

* **Wheat Bran:** Lowers blood-glucose levels and stimulates the pancreas to produce insulin.

For Cleansing the Intestinal Tract:

* **Apple Pectin:** Helps regulate the bowels and the elimination process. It also draws toxic metals out of the blood. It is said that apple pectin contains electromagnetic properties.

* **Clay:** Has the ability to absorb toxins. We want to prevent toxins from getting into the bloodstream, because once in the bloodstream, damage will result. This is especially true if the immune system and liver are not operating at absolute top efficiency.

* **Dandelion Root:** Improves liver function. Bile and certain enzymes produced in the liver aiding maintaining proper intestinal flora.

* **Flax Seed:** Provides "pushing and sweeping" benefits.

* **Marshmallow Root:** Soothes mucous membranes; used internally to treat inflammation and mucosal afflictions.

* **Psylium husks:** Act as brooms for the intestines. They provide no nutrient value, however, they push through the bulk and provide fiber that helps the body eliminate waste.

* **Slippery Elm Bark:** Effective, both internally and externally, against sore and inflamed mucous membranes.

Diverticulitis (Crohn's Disease, Irritable Bowel Syndrome, Colitis)

Diverticulitis, Crohn's Disease, IBS (Irritable Bowel Syndrome), Colitis—all of these are pretty much an irritation of the villi throughout the intestinal tract, just in different areas.

In fact, anytime you see the suffix "itis," it signifies that there is inflammation.

Across the board, there are two approaches to relief – enemas or drinking tea. In this way you are saturating from the top. You can call this approach a complete GI (gastrointestinal) saturation.

You want to use four particular herbs:

* First, marshmallow root and slippery elm bark. Both of these are wonderful for soothing irritated villi.

* Bayberry bark and white oak bark also are great astringent herbs, therefore reducing the inflammation of the villi.

Make a strong brew from the herbs and use as a tea or in an enema bag. I would put one tablespoon of each herb in about twelve ounces of boiled, distilled water. Bring the water to a boil, take it off the stove, throw in the herbs, let it steep, strain, drink and use.

If there is a rectal ulcer or duodenal or peptic ulcer, throw some cayenne into the mix and it will facilitate the healing of the ulcer.

Cayenne is wonderful for many different applications. As we have already spoken about, it is great for ulcers: a tablespoon of cayenne in a glass of warm water, mix it together and drink it before you go to bed. That should take care of a peptic or duodenal ulcer.

If you feel a heart attack coming on, you can put some cayenne under your tongue, sublingually, and that should help equalize the blood pressure. If you get severely cut, you can take cayenne and continue to throw it on the cut; it will stop the bleeding.

In the wintertime, when you are going to go out and play in the snow, put cayenne in the bottom of your shoes before you put them on. This will help keep your feet warmer.

Dysentery (See Diarrhea)

Ear Infections

Ear, nose (sinus) and throat infections, I believe, are all the same: basically a Candida flare up, because Candida is natural to the throat — it is where it lives. The reason for ear infections, sinus congestion and throat issues is because the immune system is under stress and is faltering. Because of this, the Candida is no longer held in check and, therefore, begins to flourish greatly.

In order to eliminate ear infections, use the herbs garlic, goldenseal root and/or black walnut hulls.

* **Garlic:** wonderful for ear infections. In fact, there is an old Mexican naturalist approach, which is to take a clove garlic, warm it between the hands, stick a needle and thread through it, and then insert it when it is still warm into the child's ear. The garlic obviously is an irritant. It will draw blood to the area, and then with the thread, you can pull the garlic out.

* **Black walnut:** known for eliminating parasites.

* **Goldenseal root:** another antibiotic. It can also be used as a tea, as well.

Mix the herbs in oil, ideally let them sit in the sun or gently heat to infuse the oil with the properties of the herbs. Strain, and use the oil as an eardrop.

For sinus infections, take the same herbs and make a tea and perform a nasal douche, using a neti pot for ideal application. By washing out the sinus cavities with those herbs, you kill the infection that has grown out of control.

For the throat, you can use a couple of different things: I would take the same herbal mixture, make a strong tea and mix it with honey, so that it is more of an elixir which will slowly coat the throat. You could also crush a garlic clove and add it to the mix.

There is a liquid called Loquat, which is a thick syrup of fruit extracts. It is very healing and soothing.

Emphysema (See Congestion and Sinus Problems)

Energy Problems

In my opinion, energy problems are a result of poor nutrition, overindulgence in sugar,, stress, and being overwhelmed. Energy is manufactured in the cells within the mitochondria. It requires a constant source of such fuels as fat and pantothenic acid. Pantothenic acid becomes co-enzyme A and that starts the Krebs cycle, the production of energy.

Pantothenic acid benefits the adrenal glands, which supports the body in stress. The adrenal glands also regulate sugar in the blood stream. When sugar is too high the adrenals communicate with the pancreas to secret insulin to bring the sugar down to normal levels.

When sugar gets too low, when energy gets too low, the adrenals are supposed to talk to the liver to release glycogen into the blood stream so that there is fuel for the cells. However, if the glands are spent through stress and exhausted from over-communicating with the pancreas to regulate sugar in the blood, the result is low energy.

Most people do not get enough pantothenic acid in their diet or supplements.

For a list of the nutrients to nourish the adrenal glands see the section on Chronic Fatigue.

Fibromyalgia

Medical science has no idea what causes fibromyalgia. It is as though the pain is circulating throughout the body. It may be caused by pollution; toxins aggravating nerve endings where they are pooling temporarily. Imagine it as sludge – a floating sludge – like oil balls in the Gulf of Mexico. Just imagine that you have these little sludge balls floating around, and wherever they get lodged there is pain.

Performing a detox and cleanse (see section on Detoxing) is one beneficial approach, as well as adding malic acid and magnesium immediately to your diet. In addition, I would also choose a multi-mineral and a basic foundation program based on your gender.

Fertility Problems (Male and Female)

For our survival, healthy human beings require a whole regimen of nutrients. Those nutrients come to us in the form of fresh air, clean water, sunshine, fats, carbohydrates, proteins, vitamins and minerals. Healthy thinking is also key.

Reproduction and Pregnancy

The process of reproduction, also known as "life's greatest miracle," is the process by which new individuals of a species are produced and genetic material is passed from generation to generation. Parent cells pass along material to daughter cells along the path of cell division. This very important process allows for growth and development of a fetus from a cellular level to the level of separation of a child from the mother. Of course, growth continues through childhood and into the adult cycle of life. However, the period of development in the womb and during early childhood is critical to overall health and growth into adulthood.

Changes in the body accompany pregnancy. There is an increase in blood flow and volume, an increase in body oxygen, an increase in appetite, and changes in the skin, to name but a few. With all the changes that occur, it becomes even more important to nourish the body (or bodies).

Nutrition Plays a Vital Role

Fresh air, sunshine and clean water speak for themselves. Fresh air brings in large amounts of oxygen, which helps to nourish the body. The brain uses 25% of all the oxygen in the body. Sunshine helps the body produce vitamin D, which is essential for many different nutritional and enzymatic transactions. Water, of course, plays a major role in the body's health. Without water, the body cannot perform many critical functions. Fresh air and fresh water are the essence of our continued existence as a species.

Foods provide you with fats, carbohydrates and proteins. Foods also contain vitamins, minerals and enzymes. All of these substances are necessary for good health. Research has shown that nutrition plays a major role in the reproduction function by influencing the health of fetal development.

The amounts of many vitamins and minerals needed during pregnancy and lactation are increased. The National Research Council of the National Academy of Sciences has established separate Recommended Daily Allowances for pregnant and lactating women to reflect these higher nutrient needs.

Nutritional Support for Reproduction

Nourishment for the reproductive process includes many 'do's and don'ts.' For example, the maternal use of chemicals and dangerous drugs has a potentially dangerous effect on the fetus and newborn. There is an enormous list of potentially dangerous products, so question everything you ingest. Also, common sense suggests that the dangers of smoking, drugs and drinking alcohol are multiplied by two during pregnancy. Exposure to radiation is another danger and caution is advised, especially during the first trimester of pregnancy.

Both spouses play a role in the reproductive process. For healthy procreation, it is wise for both partners to strive for healthy well-being.

Committees of experts on dietary allowances advise that there needs to be an increase in the intake of most vitamins and minerals during pregnancy and lactation. These committees all agree that maternal supplementation has, in general, a positive effect on birth weight.

Infertility Issues

It is astounding to read reports that imply there are over 2 million couples who cannot have children because of infertility problems. There are many causes for infertility in each sex, and some of the problems lie in psychological areas such as not wanting to remain in the relationship, not wanting the responsibilities or stress of parenthood, or even fearing the rigors of parenthood. Still others are conflicted by their career goals or a reluctance to take on the financial burdens of having and raising a child.

All of these psychological factors cause internal stress, and stress depletes the body's nutritional reserves. Poor nutritional reserves coupled with an inadequate diet cause even greater depletion of the essential nutrients necessary for the proper functioning of the reproductive system. With these factors in mind, one ideal approach to resolving these issues would be to replace as efficiently as possible all of the nutrients that the body would require.

Like every other condition within the human body, the inability to conceive has multiple causes. In women, two common physical causes are blocked fallopian tubes and endometriosis.

Another cause may be an allergy that the body develops toward the egg. I have seen this in gay women who are trying to conceive; usually this develops in the partner that becomes the "dominant male" of the relationship and seeks to become pregnant.

Within each human body are both female and male hormones, so people are, in essence, both female and male. In some gay women who are trying to conceive, the mind/body has difficulty because childbearing is contradictory to the concepts a gay woman maintains about herself, her identity and her sexual role. You can begin to understand why the body would attack the eggs as an alien invader. In order to protect itself, the egg would create an impenetrable shell—because all living things have an innate desire to survive and live—thus, fertilization would be difficult in this scenario.

Irregular menstrual periods in the woman may also make it difficult or impossible to predict ovulation, while male infertility factors can include a low sperm count, weak motility, or both.

In many cases of infertility, the odds for a successful conception and pregnancy can be greatly strengthened through improved nutrition.

The following information is provided to help you better understand the role that certain nutrients play in the overall health during the reproductive cycle, as well as the pregnancy and lactation processes of reproduction.

Nutrients, Amino Acids and Herbs for Male Reproductive System Support:

* **Beta-carotene (Vitamin A):** Vitamin A is a fat-soluble nutrient that plays an important role in the formation of bones, teeth and skin. It is necessary during pregnancy and lactation since fetal requirements for vitamin A increase the maternal need for it. Many experts advise a 25% increase over pre-pregnancy intake.

* **B-complex Vitamins:** Needed for two reasons: (1) B-vitamin blood levels generally decline during pregnancy, hormonal changes, and (2) fetal levels exceed those in the mother, reflecting active transport across the placenta. Studies indicate that B-6 needs tend to increase in pregnant women whose diets are rich in protein.

* **Vitamin B-1** is important for carbohydrate metabolism, digestion, and heart function.

* **Vitamin B-6** is necessary for the proper functioning of both nerves and muscles, including pressure-sensitive nerve cells and cardiac muscles.

* **Vitamin B-12** helps form normal red blood cells and a healthy nervous system, and is important for its role in DNA synthesis.

* **Folic Acid:** Necessary for growth, cell division and red blood cell formation. It helps with reproduction and is necessary for the health of the glands and liver.

* **Inositol:** Necessary for hair growth, fat and cholesterol metabolism, and lecithin formation.

* **Niacin/Niacinamide:** A B-complex nutrient that plays a role in growth and the proper functioning of the nervous system.

* **Pantothenic Acid:** Essential for growth, contributes to energy functions and is necessary for the skin.

* **Vitamin C:** Essential for the absorption of inorganic iron and strong immune system function. Plays a role in collagen production. Pregnancy increases the need for vitamin C.

* **Vitamin E:** Participates in the synthesis of hemoglobin. The motility and fertility of sperm are in proportion to the amount of vitamin E in a man's semen.

* **Calcium:** A mineral necessary for metabolism and the building of bones and teeth.

* **Iron:** Supplementation is essential for almost all pregnancies, especially for women with low serum ferritin levels.

* **Magnesium:** Plays a role in neuromuscular activity and impulse transmission.

* **Manganese:** Plays a role in enzyme activation.

* **Zinc:** Aids in the metabolism of phosphorus and protein. Zinc also participates in the metabolism of RNA.

* **L-Arginine, L-Cysteine, L-Glutamine and L-Methionine:** Amino acids that are vital to the production of sperm as well as having a healthy uterus.

* **Damiana**

* **Ginseng Root**

* **Sarsaparilla**

* **Saw Palmetto**

Nutrients and Herbs for Female Reproductive System Support:

The following should be included in the diet to support a woman's overall health during the reproductive cycle, as well as during pregnancy and lactation:

* **Beta-carotene (Vitamin A):** Vitamin A is a fat-soluble nutrient that plays an important role in the formation of bones, teeth and skin. It is necessary during pregnancy and lactation since fetal requirements for vitamin A increase the maternal need for it. Many experts advise a 25% increase over pre-pregnancy intake.

* **B-complex Vitamins:** Needed for two reasons: (1) B-vitamin blood levels generally decline during pregnancy, hormonal changes, and (2) fetal levels exceed those in the mother, reflecting active transport across the placenta. Studies indicate that B-6 needs tend to increase in pregnant women whose diets are rich in protein.

* **Vitamin B-1** is important for carbohydrate metabolism, digestion, and heart function.

* **Vitamin B-6** is necessary for the proper functioning of both nerves and muscles, including pressure-sensitive nerve cells and cardiac muscles.

* **Vitamin B-12** helps form normal red blood cells and a healthy nervous system, and is important for its role in DNA synthesis.

* **Folic Acid:** Necessary for growth, cell division and red blood cell formation. It helps with reproduction and is necessary for the health of the glands and liver.

* **Niacin/Niacinamide:** A B-complex nutrient that plays a role in growth and the proper functioning of the nervous system.

* **Pantothenic Acid:** Essential for growth, contributes to energy functions and is necessary for the skin.

* **Vitamin C:** Essential for the absorption of inorganic iron and strong immune system function. Plays a role in collagen production. Pregnancy increases the need for vitamin C.

* **Vitamin D:** Important in the reproductive cycle. Studies have shown that vitamin D plays a role in promoting positive calcium balance in pregnant women.

* **Vitamin E:** Participates in the synthesis of hemoglobin. The motility and fertility of sperm are in proportion to the amount of vitamin E in a man's semen.

* **Iron:** Supplementation is essential for almost all pregnancies, especially for women with low serum ferritin levels.

* **Zinc:** Aids in the metabolism of phosphorus and protein. Zinc also participates in the metabolism of RNA.

* **Unsaturated Fatty Acids** are essential building material for making hormones, as well as helping the body to build tissue.

* **L-Arginine, L-Cysteine, L-Glutamine and L-Methionine: Amino acids** that are vital to the production of sperm as well as having a healthy uterus.

* **Capsicum**

* **False Unicorn Root**

* **Gotu Kola**

* **Red Raspberry**

* **Wild Yam Root**

Psychological Considerations

Shaky finances, uncertainty or ambivalence about your partner or relationship, conflicting career aspirations, and a fear of the lifestyle changes and responsibilities associated with parenthood can play a part in sabotaging fertility at the subconscious level.

These are all legitimate reasons that one or both partners may have for not wanting to have a child at a particular time. Without honest discussion between the partners, these feelings may never be consciously expressed; they may only serve to block conception.

When a couple consciously wants to have a child but cannot conceive or carry a pregnancy to term, then along with any health or nutrition issues involved, it is important to look at the subconscious energies and concepts at work. Both parties must equally share in the desire to have a child.

Fungal Infections

Fungal infections have many causes. A common thread is a weakened immune system. Normally the immune system is able to hold everything at bay when you are not under stress. However, as the stress builds and the adrenal glands falter, the immune system falters with them, as well. When a person is under stress, conditions such as infections from fungi, germs, viruses, Candida, or outbreaks of herpes, shingles, acne and allergies will flare up.

Resolving fungal issues depends on where the fungus is located. We will start from the bottom and work our way up beginning with toenail funguses and/or Athlete's foot. Here are a couple of different ways to approach these problems:

* **Pau D' Arco:** is an herb that kills bacteria. In fact, it is reported that it has such antibacterial properties that no bacteria lives in the soil immediately around the roots of the tree. It is as if it has created this defense mechanism that yields a toxic dose to bacteria. We use it for the same purpose; to kill bacteria, fungus and critters of that nature.

* **Myrrh:** contains similar antibacterial properties. However, it is a resin, which can be a little bit difficult to work with.

* **Black Walnut Hulls**

* **Goldenseal Roo**t

One approach is to make a strong tea/foot bath made out of goldenseal root, Pau D' Arco, myrrh and black walnut hulls — the same as used for skin infections earlier.

A similar approach is the one used for eliminating "jungle rot" in South America. To kill fungus under the nails as well as athlete's foot, they would soak their feet in organic corn-meal mush. Interestingly, if you visit a gardening store, organic cornmeal is sold to kill lawn grubs.

Moving up the body, some may encounter vaginal infections. You can use the same tea that is used for skin and fungus as a douche and that should take care of it.

Other areas of fungal infections would be around the nostril, which more often than not is going to be a Candida overgrowth. In this situation apply the tea mixture topically. It is a wonderful combination of herbs. It would be wise to strengthen the adrenal glands and the immune system at the same time. Candida overgrowth creates thrush as well as ear infections and sinus infections. Candida lives in the throat naturally.

When the immune system is overwhelmed and undernourished, and the body is stressed, the immune system will falter and the Candida will flourish everywhere, especially in the intestinal tract, if it is there.

Gallstones

Gallstones are a misnomer; they should be called gall clumps because the "stones" are really globs of cholesterol that become clumped together in the sac-like gall bladder. Gallstones are primarily the result of too much fried food and a diet high in saturated fats. This is why the stones have a cholesterol-type base.

Below is a general process often recommended within the health food industry that can be used to dissolve gallstones:

1. Take three tablespoons of cold-pressed olive oil and one teaspoon of freshly squeezed lemon juice. Wait for fifteen minutes.

2. Repeat the process until you have consumed a small bottle of olive oil.

3. If you should happen to vomit, simply rinse your mouth with water. Do not swallow the water. Continue the process.

This entire process should be started on an empty stomach first thing in the morning. The very first bowel movement you have will contain gallstones. I have never heard of one complaint with this process, other than the taste of the olive oil. Afterward, eat a large salad. (Do not eat onions from open salad bars. Onions draw bacteria to themselves.)

Glaucoma

Glaucoma is a disease of the eyes marked by increased pressure within the eye, which soon damages the optic nerve. People with glaucoma have a tendency to be thiamine deficient.

With everything currently known about glaucoma, at least one aspect remains in question: what causes the drainage canal behind the eye to become inflamed and, therefore, blocked? The purpose of this channel, called the Schlemm's canal, is to allow the fluid within the eye, called aqueous humor, to drain. Fluid constantly enters the eye, so when a blockage occurs drainage is prevented. Pressure builds up behind the eye because none of the fluid is able to exit.

The most common type of glaucoma is open-angle. It is without symptoms in the earliest stages, producing an entirely painless increase in eyeball pressure. Peripheral vision may be slowly affected. Those with a family history of this disease are at greatest risk. African Americans, the severely nearsighted, diabetics, people over sixty-five years of age, and anyone taking hypertension drugs or cortisone carry a high risk as well.

A diet rich in vitamin A and the B complex vitamins, especially inositol, is recommended for those afflicted with the condition.

Vitamin C can help glaucoma by increasing osmotic pressure in the blood, which, in turn, pulls fluid out of the eyeball.

Another highly effective regimen is adding proteolytic enzymes. They work by eliminating malformed proteins and protein debris, which are harmful. When working with these enzymes make sure they are taken on an empty stomach and the tablets are enteric coated. That way they will dissolve in your intestinal tract, enter your blood stream and head for the damaged and inflamed areas. I know from experience in working with a client that these work for reducing inflammation anywhere in the body.

Nutrients and Herbs to Support Eye Health:

* **Vitamin A:** Essential for all vision, especially healthy night vision. Vitamin A also serves as an antioxidant. It is a potent quencher of singlet oxygen, a highly reactive molecule form or configuration believed to be responsible for aging. It breaks down DNA so that reproduced cells are flawed and weak. This leads to aging and disease.

* **Vitamin B-1:** Necessary for healthy mouth, skin, eyes and hair.

* **Vitamin B-2:** Good for cell respiration and the maintenance of good vision, skin, nails and hair.

* **Vitamin B-6:** Required for the proper absorption of vitamin B-12, the production of hydrochloric acid and magnesium assimilation.

* **Vitamin B-12:** Helps form normal red blood cells and a healthy nervous system.

* **Choline:** Part of the neurotransmitter acetylcholine, which is essential for the transmission of impulses (electrical energy) through the nervous system.

* **Folic Acid:** Another vitamin that has a direct nourishing and fortifying effect on the "frontline" of the body's defense system.

* **Inositol:** Closely associated with choline and biotin; also needed for the growth and survival of cells in bone marrow, eye membranes and intestines.

* **Niacin:** Promotes growth and proper nervous system function.

* **Pantothenic Acid:** Also known as vitamin B-5, pantothenic acid helps in the utilization of other vitamins, especially vitamin B-2.

* **Vitamin C:** Strengthens the blood vessels and also helps to detoxify the effects of heavy metals often found in drinking water, for example, lead.

* **Eyebright:** A traditional herb for eyes.

* **Ginger:** A circulatory stimulant. Considered a "packager" because it carries nutrients throughout the system.

* **Biotin**

The Proteolytic Enzymes:

Pancreatin is an enzyme secreted by the pancreas to aid in the digestive process.

Papain is an enzyme found in papaya fruit, plays a key role in the digestion of protein.

* **Trypsin** is a chromium-dependent enzyme that aids in the breakdown of amino acids for absorption.

* **Amylase** is an enzyme that works to breakdown carbohydrates. One of the more potent digestive enzymes, amylase is found in both pancreatic secretions and in saliva.

* **Lipase** is the enzyme that deals with the breakdown of fats and cholesterol in the digestive system.

* **Chymotrypsin** is a pancreatic enzyme that breaks down proteins.

Goiter (See Thyroid Problems)

Growing Pains (See Minerals)

Hair Loss (See Circulation)

Headaches (See Migraines)

Heart

The most amazing organ in the human body is the heart. It is a remarkable piece of machinery. As the center of the cardio-vascular system, the heart propels blood through thousands of miles of blood vessels, pumping more than 30 times its weight in blood each minute[70]. Even at rest, the heart pumps more than 1800 gallons of blood a day. For all the work required of the heart, it is relatively small, about the size of a closed fist.

The most incredible aspect of the heart is that it is constructed well enough to operate without a moment's rest for an entire lifetime. Humankind's most advanced technology has yet to equal such extraordinary functioning and durability.

Heart Function

The function of the heart is to adjust the body's circulation in relation to the metabolic rate of body cells. This employs the pumping action of the heart, aided by both chemical and nervous controls.

Age, gender, physical activity and body temperature all influence the heart. Heart rate is high in newborns and declines with age, although heart rate can increase among senior citizens[71]. Females generally have slightly higher heart rates than males.

Physical activity can lower resting heart rate, which is important because a slowly beating heart is more energy efficient than one that beats rapidly. Exercise is perhaps the most important factor in a properly functioning heart for several reasons. First, exercise increases the oxygen demand on the muscles. It also increases high-density lipoproteins, important for the proper distribution and elimination of cholesterol from the blood. Exercise also improves lung function, which brings more oxygen into the bloodstream. Exercise controls weight and increases endorphins, the body's natural painkillers. Finally, exercise helps make bones stronger and reduces blood pressure[72].

Nutrients for the Heart

If the heart is considered the engine of the body, then the blood must be considered the oil. Nutrition plays a key role in the functions of both, as well as the supporting organs and functions for the system. Proper nutrition is needed for the heart and allows blood to efficiently carry the nutrients necessary to feed the cells of the body.

The following nutrients play a key role in the proper functioning of the heart:

* **Calcium**: important for its essential role in such vital functions as nerve conduction, muscle contraction, blood clotting and membrane permeability[73,74]. It also plays a role in the transmission of nerve impulses, important in the function of blood pressure maintenance. Calcium ions play a role in the strength of cardiac muscular contraction, similar to skeletal muscle fiber function[75].

* **Magnesium**: important in neuromuscular activity and myocardial functioning[76]. This essential mineral also plays a role in potassium and calcium homeostasis[77].

* **Potassium:** plays a role in cardiac muscle contraction. Positive potassium ions are involved in the resting action after the beat of the heart muscle fiber, known as repolarization[78]. It also contributes to the maintenance of normal blood pressure[79].

* **Vitamin D:** essential in the maintenance of calcium homeostasis. It serves to mobilize calcium within the body, allowing it to be more readily assimilated. This is important not only to the heart functions of calcium, but for the body in general.

* **Vitamin E:** protects fat-soluble vitamins during their tenure in the body. It functions as an antioxidant and prevents the spread of the oxidation of certain fatty acids that leads

to cell structure and membrane damage[80].

* **Co q10:** prevents oxidation of LDL cholesterol. Cellular energy production supports cell membrane integrity

* **Fish oil:** helps the body regulate healthy triglyceride and cholesterol levels. It is also necessary for cell membrane integrity and the natural inflammatory process.

Heart Burn (See Acid Reflux)

Hemorrhoids (See Varicose Veins)

Hepatitis

Hepatitis is a viral disease. It attacks the liver and leads to inflammation. People infected with the virus (HCV) have no symptoms. Most people are not aware that they have the hepatitis C infection until liver damage shows up. This may be decades later during routine medical tests.

Nutritional Support

Nutrition is an excellent example of the body's synergy. The body needs a continuous and regulated supply of nutrients for normal growth, physiological functioning and health maintenance. For a workhorse organ such as the liver, it is essential that it receives and has the ability to process all the nutrients it needs and distributes to the body. The following vitamins and minerals play an important role in the functioning of the liver and the overall health of the body. Of the three (3) types of hepatitis – A, B and C – hepatitis C is the most serious. It has been successfully eliminated from individuals by utilizing the following herbs and nutrients:

* **Vitamin A** is important to the functioning of the liver. The liver utilizes beta carotene to produce vitamin A, which is stored in the liver to be used as needed.

* **Vitamin E** functions as an antioxidant and protects vitamin A and unsaturated fatty acids from oxidation. It also participates in hemoglobin synthesis and maintains cell membrane integrity.

* **Vitamin B-12** is involved in the metabolism of single carbon units which play a role in cell growth.

* **B-Complex** vitamins play an important role in liver function.

* **Vitamin B-1** participates in the process of carbohydrate metabolism within the liver and is essential in the transformation of tryptophan to niacin.

* **Niacin** is a constituent of two coenzymes involved in metabolism.

* **Pantothenic Acid** is a constituent of coenzyme A, essential for the formation of cholesterol.

* **Choline** is essential for liver function as a constituent of lecithin, a group of phosphorus-rich fats found in the liver, which are essential for transforming fats in the body.

* **Vitamin K** plays an important role in liver function as a co-factor in the liver synthesis of prothrombin and other coagulation factors[81].

* **Lecithin** is a water-dispersable fat that bonds to other fats within the body. It is a great way to break up fatty deposits within the liver and in the blood stream. As it breaks down, choline and inositol are its byproducts.

* **Milk thistle** is known for stimulating new cellular growth in the liver, which is obviously important.

* **Yellow dock** is a blood purifier more than anything else. It is also known to be good for stimulating the liver and bile production.

* **L-Methionine** is an amino acid that works with choline and inositol and helps to emulsify fats and cholesterol.

One of the things that some of the nutrients do is break up the fatty deposits in the liver. This allows for more efficient and essential chemical conversions to take place within the liver. Other nutrients such as A, C and Zinc are for the immune system and help destroy the virus and any corrupted cells.

Herpes

Herpes and shingles are of the same family. Fundamentally, it is the same virus responsible for chicken pox virus; a virus that lives at the nerve endings. 99% of the time their existence is never an issue.

When there is so much stress that the adrenal glands begin to falter and crash, they bring the immune system down with them at the same time. Therefore, everything that the immune system held at bay now has an opportunity to flourish. Herpes, shingles, acne, allergies – all of these will flare up. Candida and hypoglycemia are also tied into the adrenals.

For shingles, there are two methods you can use. One, you could put garlic oil topically on the outbreaks. I have been told by many that it seems to dry them up. You can either buy pearls or liquid garlic in oil, or make your own. Apply that topically to help dry up the open sore or irritation. Two, build the immune system (see the Immune System section). Strengthen the adrenal glands (see the nutrients listed in the Energy section).

High Blood Pressure (Hypertension)

High blood pressure, or hypertension, has many different causes. An example would be a breakdown in the communication between the nerves and the cells that comprise the heart, as well as the muscles surrounding the arterial system. The breakdown can lead to improper muscular tension and conditions that ultimately result in hypertension.

Hypertension is also the result of today's fast-paced, anxiety-filled lifestyle, which is conducive to the accumulation of stress and tension—two underlying causes of hypertension. Stress, tension and anxiety are not entirely physical diseases, although they do cause them. Instead, they are the result of emotional and mental attitudes about situations and consequent behavior towards them.

Internal reactions at emotional levels cause slight chemical reactions within the body. An excellent example of this is when the phone rings in the middle of the night. As a parent, this event will usually trigger a biochemical reaction within the individual. One such change will be a drop of calcium in the body due to shock and stress, and when calcium is compromised it creates an imbalance between sodium and potassium. This, in turn, will cause the body to retain fluid, putting pressure on the cardiovascular system and, as a result, could elevate blood pressure.

Another affect of this chemical stimulation is that the body may begin to tighten up as the muscles contract. This contraction places excessive pressure on the cardiovascular system, leading to elevated blood pressure.

Stress

If stress, either internal or external, causes an increase in heartbeat, the following sequence occurs. The heart increases its beats per minute, pushing more blood through the ventricle into the arteries at a faster rate, which increases the pressure on the walls of the arteries. This higher pressure is detected by the pressure-sensitive nerve cells in the arteries and they send messages to the brain in the form of nerve impulses. The brain responds to the message by telling the heart to slow down, which should decrease the blood pressure and defuse the situation. The nervous system continually monitors blood pressure in this manner in an effort to maintain a normal flow of blood. This is called a feedback system.

A feedback system is any circular situation in which information and the status of an operation are continually reported to a central control area. The manner in which the nervous system and the brain interact is a good example of a feedback system. For this feedback system to function properly and maintain the homeostasis of the body, the different elements of the systems involved must be in proper working order. The blood vessels, the nerve cells and the brain's neurotransmitters must all function together to maintain the homeostasis of the blood pressure.

Nutrients, Amino Acids and Herbs to Support Normal Blood Pressure

There are many dangers to uncontrolled high blood pressure. Stroke and death are two of these dangers. Include the following in your diet to help reduce high blood pressure through the elimination of excess water, muscular tension and vasodilatation.

* **Calcium:** Important for neuromuscular excitability and the transmission of nerve impulses.

* **Magnesium:** Acts as an electrolyte along with calcium and potassium.

* **Potassium:** Works along with vitamin B-6 in maintaining proper water balance. Often, an imbalance in osmosis creates pressure on the arterial system.

* **Vitamin B-6:** Aids in maintaining correct water balance in the blood and tissues. It is necessary for the proper function of the pressure-sensitive nerve cells and cardiac muscles important in the body's normal blood pressure homeostasis.

* **Vitamin D:** Ensures the effectiveness of calcium.

* **L-Taurine:** A free-form amino acid known to affect certain biological functions, including cardiac contractility, and as a mood enhancer.

* **Apple Pectin, Cayenne, and Garlic:** All have the ability to equalize blood pressure.

* **Hawthorne Berries:** Tone and strengthen the heart muscle.

* **Hops and Valerian Root:** Calming herbs to the nervous system.

High Cholesterol and Triglycerides

One cause of high cholesterol could be a faulty liver and over-production of cholesterol. More often than not, high cholesterol is the direct result of the diet. Americans eat too much sugar and sweeteners in just about everything. In addition to the sugars, there is also the consumption of saturated, hydrogenated and trans fats in the diet. Alcohol also affects the health of the liver. All of these elements cause the liver to become fatty and, therefore, impede its performance, especially in the arena of detoxifying.

High cholesterol and triglycerides cause thickening of the blood as well as contributing to hardening of the arteries.

Cholesterol is a Fat

Fats, medically and nutritionally referred to as lipids, are essential for good health. Triglycerides, also known as neutral fats, act as a source of insulation, protection, source of energy and major energy storage molecules in the body. Phospholipids, fats that contain phosphorus, are the major lipid component of cell membranes and are found in high amounts in the brain and nerve tissues.

The Importance of Fats

A fat is a substance containing one or more fatty acids that is the principle form in which energy is stored in the body[82,83]. A certain amount of fat is necessary in the diet to provide an adequate supply of essential fatty acids to the body and for the efficient absorption of fat-soluble vitamins from the intestine(84). A surplus of carbohydrates, proteins or fats in the diet are all converted to triglycerides and stored in fat tissue[85].

Metabolism of Fats

Metabolism is the term used to describe the chemical and physical changes that take place within the body that enable it to grow and function[86]. Fat metabolism is related to basal metabolism; that is, the "base" rate of chemical reactions occurring within the body while it is at rest[87].

Metabolism of Fats and Cholesterol

The healthy metabolism of fats, carbohydrates and proteins is one of the most important aspects of good health. There are two main types of metabolism: building up, known as anabolism, and breaking down, known as catabolism.

In anabolism, smaller molecules, such as amino acids, are converted into larger molecules, such as proteins. In catabolism the opposite is true. Larger molecules, such as glycogen, are broken down to smaller molecules, such as glucose.

It is important that cholesterol is metabolized on a continual basis. Cholesterol serves different functions in the body. It is a component of cell membranes and starting material for synthesizing other steroids. The adrenals use cholesterol as a precursor for steroid hormone production. In fact, all steroid hormones in the human body are derived from cholesterol. Cholesterol is also a precursor of vitamin D.

Essential Fatty Acids

Most triglycerides contain more than one kind of fatty acid, polyunsaturated (PUFA), saturated and mono-saturated, and most food fats are mixtures of different triglycerides[88]. The body has a specific need for PUFA since they cannot be synthesized in the body. Linoleic acid is the PUFA needed for healthy cell membranes and serves as a precursor for the formation of other fatty acids necessary within the body. Arachidonic acid is the PUFA that is a major precursor for prostaglandins, a group of chemically active, hormone-like compounds that influence innumerable body processes[89].

Nutritional Support

The following information is provided to help you better understand the role that certain nutrients play in the metabolism of cholesterol and other fats and the overall health of the body. Those nutrients are:

* **Vitamin B-6** is necessary for the metabolism of fats-carbohydrates-proteins.

* **Choline** is important to the metabolism and transport of fats and cholesterol and in the formation of lecithin.

* **Inositol** is used in the metabolism of fats and cholesterol and in the formation of lecithin.

* **Niacin** is another nutrient necessary for the metabolism of fats, carbohydrates and proteins.

* **Pantothenic Acid** is necessary for growth, contributing to energy functions, and to the skin.

* **Chromium** is essential for the production of insulin, used by the body to regulate cholesterol production.

* **Iodine** is an essential part of the hormones thyroxine and triiodothyronine.

* **Magnesium** is essential for the normal metabolism of potassium and calcium.

* **Zinc** is also involved in the production of insulin.

* **Unsaturated Fatty Acids** are essential for growth.

Hyperactivity

Hyperactivity can have different causes, from artificial flavoring and colors to too much caffeine and sugar. All of those are contributing factors along with emotional components and genetic considerations.

What needs to be done nutritionally, first and foremost, would be utilizing the memory nutrients (see the Memory section), as well as the nerve nutrients for calming. The memory nutrients will open up the mind to nourish the brain and to make for better synapses. Also, with hyperactivity, a substance not in any of the nutrients recommended above, but one specifically for hyperactivity, would be Guarana. It works the same as Ritalin. It helps balance out the brain. Though I have not had any personal experience with this, it comes highly recommended from a grandmother who cares dearly for her grandchildren. (See Nerve section. See also Stress and Tension section.)

Hypoglycemia (Low Blood Sugar)

Hypoglycemia is the medical term for low blood sugar, and is generally caused by poor dietary habits and/or excessive of stress. It is surprising how many people constantly feel tired and run down, even after a full night's sleep. Are you in this group, or do you know someone who is? Chronic tiredness—even after sleeping up to 12 hours a night—is perhaps the most identifiable of hypoglycemia's symptoms, which also include irritability, depression and headaches.

Hypoglycemics are the kind of people you do not talk to until you give them something to eat or drink in the morning to raise their blood sugar level. However, nourishing the adrenals is a much better solution, as it will address the physical aspects. Pantothenic acid, vitamin C and a little dash of licorice root strengthen the adrenals so there is good communication with the liver.

Many people try to deal with this problem by taking B-12 injections, the mineral chromium or stimulant herbs high in caffeine, such as Guarana or Ephedra (Ma Huang). This approach is not the answer. It is only a form of relief without addressing the true cause. These herbs work by stimulating the central nervous system, which is an unhealthy approach to the problem. The proper approach lies in good nutrition and dietary changes.

Knowing how difficult it is to change eating habits, I have researched and found the nutritional elements that will help the body to correct hypoglycemia. First, let us examine how low blood sugar occurs. As we stated, one cause of low blood sugar is brought about by stress, and when the body is subjected to stressful conditions, it depletes the fuel supply, and so more fuel must then be added to the system.

The adrenal glands are involved with blood sugar regulation. They tell the pancreas when to start and stop insulin production. Insulin (a hormone produced by the pancreas to regulate the blood glucose level) is used to shuttle blood sugar into the cells. When too many refined carbohydrates are eaten requiring constant communication from the adrenals to the pancreas, exhaustion can begin to set in.

The adrenal glands generally are communicating with the pancreas throughout the day. By 3:00 p.m. they are exhausted from telling the pancreas to start and stop insulin production, and the last message that the pancreas received was to start insulin production. As insulin production continues blood sugar levels decrease. When blood sugar levels are low it is the responsibility of the adrenal glands to signal the liver to release glycogen (blood sugar) into the bloodstream. However, because the adrenals have been talking to the pancreas all day, it cannot talk to the liver and sugar levels continue to plunge causing hypoglycemia.

Nutrients and Herbs to Support the Adrenals in Energy Production:

* **Folic Acid:** Folic acid's metabolic role is interdependent with B-12 and both are required for cell growth and repro-duction in the body and to ensure that anemia is corrected and/or prevented.

* **Pantothenic Acid:** Pantothenic acid, through chemical transactions, becomes co-enzyme A, which stimulates the Krebs cycle in the mitochondria to produce energy for the body. Also excellent for the adrenal glands.

* **Vitamin B-12:** Has been used by the medical profession for years to provide energy to tired and run down individu-als. Vitamin B-12 is a water-soluble vitamin necessary for the synthesis of nucleic acids (RNA and DNA), the main-tenance of myelin in the nervous system and the proper functioning of folic acid.

* **Vitamin C** occurs in large concentrations in both parts of the adrenal gland. It is essential in the production of the two active hormones epinephrine and norepineph-rine by the adrenal medulla. Even though the adrenals are rich in vitamin C, upon secretion of corticosteroids, large amounts of vitamin C are lost from them.

* **Aspartic Acid:** Helps to increase stamina and endurance, as well as resistance to fatigue.

* **Eleuthero Root:** Has been used for centuries as a tonic and is highly invigorating.

* **Gotu Kola:** Feeds and stimulates the brain as well as the body, and creates alertness.

* **Licorice Root:** Nourishes the adrenal glands.

Hysterectomy

Obviously, there is nothing that can be done about a hysterectomy. The reason I list it is because of the menopause issues.

Estrogen can still be produced via the adrenal glands, provided you are not taking statin-based drugs or red yeast rice. They both impede the liver from manufacturing human cholesterol, which is essential as the precursor to your hormones, as well as Vitamin D. Take a look at the Menopause and Adrenal sections for more information on how you can still eliminate night sweats and hot flashes.

Incontinence

More often than not, incontinence will be the result of a lack of muscular control. All muscular transactions are facilitated with minerals. Minerals allow the energy of thought, whether it is a conscious decision or an unconscious directive, to communicate with all of the cells that make up the muscles, so that they know to either maintain contraction or relax.

Calcium is the main mineral for contractions and magnesium for relaxation. Because of all the transactions that minerals are involved with, I would look for a separate mineral to take at night before going to bed. (See Minerals).

Indigestion

Indigestion can have many different causes, but vitamin deficiency is most often the culprit. Vitamins, especially the B complex group, are technically designated as co-enzymes because they are part of the components necessary to create enzymes in the body, such as protease, amylase and lipase.

The B vitamins are water-dispersible, meaning they easily wash out of the body. Because they are also coenzymes and used in thousands, if not millions, of different transactions in the body, there needs to be more than an adequate amount for the body to maintain health.

It is vital to have a high potency vitamin complex to ensure that all the essential transactions will take place throughout the body. When vitamin levels are low, then certain processes will not be complete and health is compromised.

Before buying a digestive enzyme, I would start off with examining my daily multivitamin. If it was not a high potency combination I would seek out a better formula so I had more B vitamins available to me. I would fix my adrenals with higher amounts of pantothenic acid, which also becomes betaine hydrochloride, a digestive enzyme.

If needed, I would take a digestive enzyme that contained some of the following nutrients:

* **Pancreatin:** an enzyme secreted by the pancreas to aid in the digestive process.

* **Papain:** an enzyme found in papaya fruit, plays a key role in the digestion of protein.

* **Trypsin:** a chromium-dependent enzyme which aids in the breakdown of amino acids for absorption.

* **Amylase:** an enzyme that works to break down carbohydrates. One of the more potent digestive enzymes, amylase is found in both pancreatic secretions and in saliva.

* **Lipase:** the enzyme that deals with the breakdown of fats and cholesterol in the digestive system.

* **Chymotrypsin:** a pancreatic enzyme that breaks down proteins.

Immune Boosting

The Immune System

Perhaps the most incredible system in the human body is the immune system. It has the task of keeping the body healthy by fighting pathogens, disease-producing microorganisms, and neutralizing their toxins. The immune system employs the skin, urine and other natural means of waste disposal in its function of keeping the body free of toxins/pathogens. Should bacteria enter the body, the immune system recruits cells in the body to fight invading bacteria and to prevent its spread.

Basic Immunology

The immune system reacts to invasion by foreign matter in several ways. In one method, the T-cells directly attack the foreign matter. This is usually an attack directed at intracellular pathogens, viruses and tissue transplants. Another mode of attack involves the B-cells. In this scenario, they are transformed into plasma cells, which manufacture and deploy antibodies. Antibodies bind together and deactivate extracellular pathogens, such as bacteria and antigens dissolved into the body's fluids[90].

By circulating both B and T cells throughout the body, intruders and other abnormal cells are destroyed or neutralized and thereby eliminated from the body. The lymphocyte cells are the basis of the body's two closely allied immune responses, both triggered by antigens[91].

Macrophages also play a major role in acquired cell-mediated immunity. These phagocyte cells are activated and mobilized by T-cells to the site of infection where they kill invading micro-organisms. Macrophages can also function in processing and presenting antigens to lymphocytes to neutralize[92].

Immune System Memory

Amazingly, certain T-cells are specifically targeted for certain types of pathogens and are termed memory cells, which remember former attacks of specific pathogens. The memory cells group together to propel a second response to a recurring pathogen, reacting quicker and stronger than the T-cells of the primary response, even decades later! This second response is usually so fast that the pathogens are destroyed before any outward signs of disease occur[93]. The immune system also has the amazing ability to distinguish between harmful matter and beneficial elements, such as nutrients.

Immune System Homeostasis

While the immune system works constantly to keep the body free from infection, there are periods of time when the body experiences a good deal of stress. Physical stress can cause the consumption of many nutrients that may directly affect immune competence. That is one of the reasons it is important the body remains well-nourished and in homeostasis.

Nutritional Support

For the complex operation of keeping the body free of toxins and invasion of microbes, the immune system requires a constant source of nutrients. Nutrients are essential for the proper growth of T-cells and B-cells, as well as the proper manufacturing of plasma and antibodies.

Fortunately, the immune system has some help in its toiling. The lymphatic system contains several important structures and organs, as well as bone marrow, which is the site of lymphocyte (both T and B cell) production. Both the lymphatic and immune systems are involved in the body's war on foreign invaders. Since these systems are a complex interplay of many cell types and chemical functions, it is not surprising that poor nutrition can influence immune response[94]. When you try to maintain good health but do not have all the right nutrients or proper amounts, you will not have a sound and healthy immune system.

To reiterate, the two causes of a weak and ineffective immune system are stress and poor nutrition. Stress is a perception and attitude problem that requires a particular form of adjustment, whereas nutrition is a dietary and supplementation adjustment. With regard to the dietary changes, the most obvious would be to include more fresh fruits and raw vegetables. More specifically, increasing garlic, onions, celery, watercress and carrots would be especially helpful, and decreasing all fried and fatty foods along with curtailing the amount of meat, fish and fowl that you eat would also be wise.

Nutrients and Herbs to Improve Resistance to Stress and Infection:

* **Vitamin A:** Helps mature antibodies in the thymus gland and protects all mucus membranes exposed to the environment. It is important in the immune system for the healthy formation of mucous membranes, part of the body's outer protection against foreign toxins. The membranes release mucus in the linings of the mouth and nose, the digestive tube and the breathing passages.

* **Folic Acid:** Involved in the formation of white blood cells and lymphocytes, the front line soldiers of the immune system.

* **Magnesium:** Activates more enzymes in the body than any other mineral. Lack of magnesium may be a contributing factor towards the development of leukemia, or cancer of the blood.

* **Pantothenic Acid:** Stimulates the adrenal glands and increases production of cortisone and other adrenal hor-

mones; can improve the body's ability to withstand stressful conditions. Pantothenic acid has been demonstrated to enhance the activity of macrophages and natural killer cells in the body. It is necessary for antibody production, part of the humoral branch of the immune system.

* **Selenium:** Appears to prevent certain kinds of cancer.

* **Vitamin B-2:** Protects cellular respiration.

* **Vitamin B-6:** Must be present for the production of antibodies and red blood cells; improves T-cell levels and mitogen stimulation.

* **Vitamin C:** Fights bacterial infections and reduces the effects on the body of some allergy-producing substances.

* Vitamin E: Prevents saturated fatty acids and vitamin A from breaking down and combining with other substances that may become harmful to the body. The B vitamins and ascorbic acid are also protected against oxidation when vitamin E is present in the digestive tract.

* **Zinc:** Essentially "mobilizes" vitamin A from the liver, so that it can perform its usual bodily functions. Protects the immune system and supports the T-cells. When zinc intake is decreased, the thymus atrophies.

* **Astragalus:** Increases in phagocytosis, interferon and cancer survival.

* **Reishi Mushroom:** Increases phagocytosis, macrophage and cell-mediated immunity; suppresses tumor growth in mice.

* **Shiitake Mushroom:** For the immune system.

* **Beta 1,3 Glucan**

* **IP6**

* **Larch (Arabinogalactin)**

Impotence

In today's high-stress world, we often find ourselves unable to perform in life as we once did. This applies to all aspects of life. However, one of the most frustrating areas is sexual expression.

The causes go beyond simple stress. For example, in some instances a person may have poor circulation. Others deal with diabetes or side effects from medication, and some suffer from psychological causes.

There is an herb that has been in use for centuries to assist man in maintaining his "nature." This herb, often taken in tablet or capsule form or as a tea, is called yohimbe. Yohimbine, the chemical within yohimbe, is a mild serotonin inhibitor. Increased serotonin levels in the brain are another possible cause of impotence. Normally, there are no undesirable after-effects with yohimbe. Individuals with sensitive stomachs may experience some queasiness or mild nausea for a few minutes shortly after drinking the tea, so it is best to sip it slowly. Persons suffering from blood pressure disorders, diabetes, hypoglycemia, active ailments, or injury of kidneys, liver or heart should not use yohimbe. In addition, yohimbe is a brief-acting monoamine oxidase inhibitor and should not be used by persons under the influence of alcohol, amphetamines (even diet pills), antihistamines, narcotics and certain tranquilizers.

Yohimbe works directly on the sex center of the brain, as well as other organs. It has been found to be very effective in re-establishing sexual relationships and is safe for both men and women.

Note: Psychological counseling is highly recommended, as most impotence problems arise from feelings of inadequacy and are often reinforced through assertive/successful mates.

Nutrients and Herbs to Remedy Impotence:

* **Zinc:** Nourishes the prostate gland and is important in sperm production.

* **Ginseng, Dong Quai, and Damiana:** All famous for their aphrodisiac properties.

* **Yohimbe Bark:** Contains yohimbine, a strong sexual stimulant. Also used as a general tonic. It can also be used by women.

Insomnia

Insomnia has many causes, such as too many stimulants like caffeine or a side effect from drugs. Whatever the cause, it prevents a full night's sleep. There are a couple of different ways to resolve the issue.

First in my mind is always a complete multi-mineral, not just calcium or a calcium/magnesium combination, but rather a combination that includes everything – zinc, iron, phosphorus and potassium to mention a few. All of those and the other minerals need to be in the product. You want to make sure that you get anywhere from 1000 to 1500 mgs of calcium at night. Let the calcium be your guide, and everything else will fall into good ratios thereafter.

Another type of combination would be minerals and herbs. The mineral component would be limited; however, nervine herbs enhance the results. These types of specialty products are different. Some may even be time-released.

Take your minerals about one-half hour to forty-five minutes before you go to bed. You will sleep well and when you wake up in the morning you will not feel drugged. (See Minerals).

Intestinal Cleanser

The need for fitness in the intestinal tract cannot be emphasized enough. Like the importance of the other cleansing organs, it is imperative to excellent health that this particular system be free of mucus and other factors that have a tendency to clog the villi.

The villi, which look like little fingers, have openings where nutrients are absorbed into the bloodstream. If the villi are clogged for any reason, the amount of nutrients that should be entering into the blood and providing food for the cells is diminished.

The body does not know what it is bringing into the bloodstream; it only knows that it should be absorbing anything that is available to it. With this in mind, it becomes important to remove all the harmful pollutants that are in the intestines as quickly as possible. The sooner that is done, the quicker the body can respond to the nutrients that are available to it.

Herbs to Assist the Body in Intestinal Cleansing:

* **Apple Pectin:** Used for its electromagnetic properties to draw out metals to be excreted through defecation.

* **Butternut Root Bark:** For its mild laxative property.

* **Dandelion Root:** Works on stimulating the liver, which protects the body by encasing toxins in fat.

* **Flax Seeds, Psyllium Husks and Rice Bran:** Offer fiber to push bulk through and to help absorb toxins.

* **Marshmallow Root and Slippery Elm Bark:** Because of their slick adhesiveness, they coat the lower bowels with a nutritious substance that strengthens and heals.

* **Pumpkin Seeds:** Kills bodily parasites.

* **Probiotics:** Your friendly intestinal bacteria that consistently need to be replaced. By having an abundance of pro-

biotics within the intestinal tract you create a hostile environment for Candida. Candida flourishes in the absence of healthy intestinal flora. (See the Candida Albicans section for more information).

Irritable Bowel Syndrome (See also Crohn's Disease)

There are many different reasons for irritable bowel syndrome, diverticulitis, colitis and crohn's disease; however, they are all similar in that the villi become highly inflamed. One treatment is an enema containing a tablespoon each of white oak bark, bayberry bark, marshmallow root and slippery elm. Bring about 12 to 14 ounces of distilled water to a boil, remove from heat, add in the herbs, let them steep, drain and use as an enema, or as a tea for diverticulitis. Ideally, the white oak bark and the slippery elm will both reduce any inflammation to the villi. Slippery elm and marshmallow root are both calming and soothing to the inflamed villi.

Kidney Cleanser

The kidneys filter the bloodstream and extract the toxins for elimination. There is a chance that calcium and certain forms of pollution may accumulate in the kidneys, and they may have to work overtime to keep the bloodstream free from reabsorbing the toxins made water soluble by the liver.

Herbs to Assist Your Body in Keeping the Kidneys Clean and Regaining Nutritional Balance:

As you feed your body organic foods and natural supplements you will see the following results. The supplements will assist the body in dissolving calcium deposits and neutralizing the acidity of the blood.

* **Buchu Leaf:** Urinary disinfectant; mildly diuretic. It is used mainly for diseases of the kidney, urinary tract and prostate.

* **Celery Seeds:** Aids and stimulates diuretic activity.

* **Hydrangea:** Used for bladder and kidney disorders, including kidney stones, inflammation and backache from kidney trouble.

* **Juniper Berries:** Works directly on the kidneys as a diuretic.

* **Parsley:** A wonderful diuretic.

* **Uva Ursi:** Has disinfectant properties and acts as an antiseptic in the urinary tract. It is also used for bladder inflammation, kidney inflammation and kidney stones.

Kidney Infections and Stones

When we talk about the kidneys, the most obvious conditions to examine are kidney infections and kidney stones. Your kidneys are a filtering device that helps you maintain proper ratios of nutrients. They protect the body by retaining the vitamins, minerals and amino acids that are required for proper system function. However, there are biochemical reasons why calcium would become lodged and grow into a stone.

Kidney infections can have many different causes. Nonetheless, the treatment for the infections is rather simple. Many people take cranberry as a way of dealing with them. Cranberry is good because it prevents the bacteria from adhering to the urethra walls.

To eliminate a kidney infection, or any type of infection in the body, the following nutrients and herbs are essential:

* **Vitamin A:** A fat-soluble nutrient that is important for the healthy function of the thymus gland, in addition to other systems in the body. The thymus is very active in the production of antibodies.

* **Vitamin C:** Stimulates immune response. It also has a generally positive effect on the common cold germs and neutralizes them.

* **Zinc:** Is essential as it seems, to "mobilize" vitamin A from the liver so that it can perform its usual bodily functions. Protects the immune system and supports the T-cells. This is very important in the production of antibodies.

* **Echinacea:** Induces living cells to excrete more interferon, which the cells already manufacture. It destroys the germs of infection directly, and bolsters the body's defenses by magnifying the white blood cell count. It protects cells against virus-related diseases, such as herpes, influenza, canker sores, etc. Has the ability to stimulate T-cell activity.

* **Garlic:** Has been proven to increase resistance against bacterial infection.

* **Goldenseal Root:** Known to contain natural properties that kill bacteria.

To dissolve kidney stones the following nutrients and herbs are highly effective:

* **Magnesium:** 1200 to 1600 mgs

* **Vitamin D:** 1000 IU water dispersible each time you take magnesium

* **Gravel Root** (whatever you can find)

In this particular instance you may want to divide the suggested supplements into four times a day.

Laryngitis

Laryngitis is an infection of the voice box resulting in sore throat. Here are some of the things you can do to kill the infection – look to Vitamins A and C, zinc and pantothenic acid as support for the adrenal glands (because when they are taxed, the immune system is also taxed).

You can also use garlic. Crush some cloves of garlic, put it on a teaspoon with honey, and slowly bring that into the throat, allowing it to sit there as long as possible. The garlic is burning and irritating, which will draw blood to the throat area, maybe even to the voice box. In that way, you bring healing nutrients of the immune system and carry away debris. Loquat is also good for the throat.

You may also want to directly enhance your immune system with the nutrients listed in the Kidney Stones section.

Leg Aches

Leg aches have diverse causes. For example, a person could have suffered an injury and that would be the cause. However, leg aches are most often the result of a lack of minerals within the system.

The role of minerals within the body is very similar to the function of light switches within the home. Minerals are catalysts, and as such they allow biological transactions to take place. Using our analogy of the light switches, they allow the energy of thought, which is converted into electricity, to travel through the nervous system and make the leap from nerve ending to receptor site on a muscle.

When there is not an adequate amount of certain minerals within the body then the electrical energy cannot make that connection. Therefore, the muscles will either be flaccid (relaxed) or they will cramp. The cramping is the muscle contracting without the message to relax, and this is the beginning of the leg aches.

The minerals that are required for proper operation and communication are calcium, magnesium, phosphorus and potassium. These are instrumental in the body's ability to contract and relax muscles.

Leg aches, "charley horses," restless leg syndrome, tossing and turning in bed, having a hard time falling asleep, PMS cramps and growing pains are an indication that the body is compromised in the areas of calcium, magnesium and potassium.

Nutrients to Help Alleviate Leg Aches:

* **Calcium:** A mineral involved in neuromuscular excitability and transmission of nerve impulses. When calcium levels in the blood are low, symptoms of increased neuromuscular irritability, seizures and cardiac cramps are possible.

* **Magnesium:** Deficiency symptoms include muscle fasciculation, tremors and spasms.

* **Potassium:** Necessary to stimulate nerve endings for muscle contractions.

* **Vitamin D:** Needs to be present for the assimilation and utilization of calcium.

Liver

Like the kidneys, the liver is a crucial organ for the body. The liver performs vital functions, the most important being the creation of glycogen. Glycogen becomes glucose, the sugar that the cells use as food, and the entire human structure requires sugar as fuel.

The next vital function is to render harmless any manmade chemical structure that is not natural to the body. If something is identified as an alien invader, the immune system attacks immediately and the liver becomes involved as the blood passes through. The detoxification process kicks in and the liver stores the toxins in fat cells as "prisoners." In this way they cannot harm the larger population of cells.

The liver is adversely affected and placed in a stressful situation by fried foods, heavy consumption of fatty foods (including meats), alcohol, smoking, and living and/or working in a polluted environment.

When the liver is cleansed it functions better, which helps the digestive and eliminative system to perform more efficiently, too. This helps in the elimination of toxic material from the body. The liver is also tied into the kidneys by processing the toxins into water-disposable products. That way, the kidneys can work with the material to get it out of the body.

Nutrients to Assist the Body in Detoxifying the Liver:

* **Choline and Inositol:** These two nutrients are often found together and are considered lipo-tropic vitamins; translated simply – fat burners. In this program they are used to break up and dissolve fatty deposits in the liver.

* **Lecithin:** Keeps cholesterol more soluble, detoxifies the liver and increases resistance to disease by helping the thymus gland carry out its functions.

* **Chicory:** Has properties very similar to dandelion. It is often used to alleviate jaundice and spleen problems. It promotes the production of bile, release of gallstones and elimination of excessive internal mucus.

* **Dandelion Root:** Stimulates liver activity, encouraging the elimination of toxins from the blood. It stimulates the flow of bile and excretion of urea. Successfully used with hepatitis, swelling of the liver, jaundice, and dyspepsia with deficient bile secretion.

Lungs

Respiratory Resistance

The normal flow of air through the lungs meets little resistance. Any condition that obstructs the air passageways increases resistance and more pressure is required to force air through. During a forced expiration, as in coughing, straining or playing a wind instrument, intrapleural pressure may increase from its normally subatmospheric (negative) value to a positive one. This greatly increases airway resistance because it results in compression of the airways.

Seldom thought of as organs of expression, the lungs are actually responsible for the force behind a few methods of exhibiting emotions. Laughing, yawning, sighing and sobbing all get their start in the respiratory system. Known as modified respiratory movements, they also include specialized forced actions such as coughing, sneezing and hiccupping. In fact, laughing and crying are the same basic movements—sometimes indistinguishable—but the rhythm of the movements and the facial expressions usually differ. The spasmodic contractions of coughing and sneezing win the expiration power play with speeds sometimes exceeding 60mph and 100mph respectively.

Respiration and Homeostasis

Your body's cells continuously use oxygen for the metabolic reactions that release energy from nutrient molecules and produce ATP, the substance that provides energy for cellular activity. At the same time, these reactions release carbon dioxide, which must be eliminated from the body because, in excess, it is toxic to cells. The cardiovascular system and the respiratory system participate equally in achieving this end. Failure of either system has the same effect on the body: disruption of homeostasis and rapid death of cells from oxygen starvation and buildup of waste products.

Homeostasis is defined as balance and harmony within the body. It is a condition created when each cell in the body functions in an internal environment that remains within certain physiological limits. This condition is not a static state; rather it is through continuous physiological adjustments that the body is able to retain this stability.

Homeostasis can be achieved when the body: 1) has the proper amounts of gases, nutrients, ions and water; 2) maintains the optimal internal temperature; and 3) has an optimal fluid volume for the health of cells. When homeostasis is disturbed, illness may result.

Nutritional Needs

It is quite obvious that the lungs depend upon muscular action in order to function properly. The act of respiration also requires proper nerve transmissions. This is all in keeping with the body's internal feedback systems. The ultimate goal of the respiratory system is to maintain the proper levels of carbon dioxide and oxygen, and the system is highly responsive to changes in the blood levels of either.

The nutrients and herbs that play a role in proper nerve and muscle function are:

* **Calcium:** essential for the function of nerves and muscles[95].

* **Vitamin D:** intake affects the absorption efficiency for calcium in the intestine[96].

* **Magnesium:** involved in many enzymatic reactions in intermediary metabolism, including the contractibility of cardiac muscles, and is essential for calcium transport and utilization[97].

* **Iron:** as a component of hemoglobin, is essential in the transportation of oxygen.

* **Vitamin B-6** is necessary for normal neurologic function[98].

* **Slippery Elm Bark**

* **Mullein**

* **Fenugreek**

* **Wind Root**

* **Horehound**

* **Gotu Kola**

Lymphatic System

The lymphatic system is a vast, complex network of capillaries, thin vessels, valves, ducts, nodes and specialized organs[99]. The system contains fluid called lymph that flows within lymphatic vessels, several structures and organs that contain lymphatic tissue, and bone marrow, the site of lymphocyte (white blood cells) production[100].

The system helps to protect and maintain the fluid environment of the body by producing, filtering and conveying lymph and by producing various blood cells[101]. The primary lymphatic organs of the body are the thymus gland and bone marrow, as they are the sites of T (thymus derived) and B (bone marrow derived) cell production[102].

The thymus gland, spleen, lymph nodes and tonsils are all referred to as lymphatic tissue; that is, they contain numerous lymphocytes. Lymphatic tissue is actually a specialized form of reticular connective tissue that carries out immune responses[103].

By circulating certain types of lymphocytes, such as T cells and B cells, throughout the body, intruders and other abnormal cells are destroyed or neutralized and eliminated from the body[104]. In addition to being a member of the lymphatic system, the thymus is also considered the "power seat" of the immune system.

Macular Degeneration

There are a couple different types of macular degeneration. Some, such as a rip in the eye, can only be addressed surgically.

There is another type where metallic ions get caught between nerve ending and receptor site so that the electric energy is not transmitted. Because it is not transmitted, there is a blank there, so that the picture you look at, which is converted into electrical energy so the mind can reconstruct it; where there are those blackouts, those are the black spots that people see. This is because of the ions blocking connection. Amino acids will take that away because amino acids chelate to metallic ions in order to help the body utilize them more effectively.

Thus the amino acids I have included in the nutrients section below are designed to remove those ions so that macular degeneration may be resolved.

Nutrients and Herbs Against Macular Degeneration:

*   **Vitamin A** contributes to the health of nearly every tissue in the body, and its role in vision is well understood. A modified, light-receptive form of vitamin A, known as 11-cis-retinol, allows a humans to see in very low light.

*   **Vitamin E**, with its antioxidant properties, maintains eye health. It interacts well with vitamin A and is necessary for epithelial health. The function of the epithalamus, located in the brain's thalamus, is to pass on nerve signals for the senses and movement.

*   **B Complex** nutrients are required for the maintenance of ocular tissue and, in particular, the cornea and optic nerve.

*   **Niacin** is a B-complex nutrient necessary for growth, the proper functioning of the nervous system, and the transmission of impulses to the body's senses.

Other nutrients, while not directly associated with ocular health, contribute to the overall health of the body. This, in turn, may affect the health and well-being of the sensory functions. Some of these nutrients include:

*   **Vitamin D** is very important because it participates in healthy bone structure and muscular development.

* **Vitamin C** has many uses in the body. It increases the absorption of iron, helps in the production of collagen, and is essential for the immune system.

* **Eyebright** has a long tradition of being helpful to all aspects of vision and eye health.

* **Ginger Root** is known to be a great "packager" of nutrients for better delivery.

* **L-Glycine, L-Glutamine, L-Arginine and L-Cysteine** are amino acids that help chelate minerals.

* **Pantothenic Acid**

* **Bioflavonoids**

* **Bilberry**

* **Bromelain**

* **L-Glutathione** (Caution: Should not be taken by pregnant or lactating women)

Male Menopause

Menopause is a naturally occurring phenomenon happening to both men and women. In men, the transition is called "the male climacteric." Most men, however, begin to exhibit slowly decreasing sexual functions in their late forties or fifties, and one study has shown that the average age for terminating inter-sexual relations was sixty-eight, though variation was great. This decline is related to decrease in testosterone secretion.

In order to keep testosterone levels normal the following nutrients and herbs are essential:

* **Vitamin C:** Humans are one of only a few species known to require a dietary source of ascorbic acid. Vitamin C functions as an antioxidant in numerous reactions in the body, and as a co-enzyme. It serves many metabolic roles.

Vitamin C has a co-enzymatic function in the metabolism of amino acids and the biosynthesis of steroid hormones, such as testosterone[105].

* **Niacin:** Niacin is a generic term for two similar compounds; nicotinic acid and nicotinamide. A B-vitamin that is intimately involved in metabolic reactions throughout the entire body, niacin participates in the breakdown of glucose for energy and in the synthesis of fat and cholesterol[106]. Cholesterol is the raw material used for testosterone production.

* **Vitamin B-6:** The active form of B-6 is pyridoxal phosphate, which is involved in a variety of reactions important to amino acid metabolism, including the conversion of tryptophan to niacinamide[107].

* **Pantothenic Acid:** The primary role of pantothenic acid is as a constituent of co-enzyme A and, as such, it is essential to many areas of cellular metabolism. Co-enzyme A is involved as an acceptor acetate group for amino acids, vitamins and sulfonamides, and also plays a role in the synthesis of cholesterol, phospholipids, steroid hormones and choline[108].

* **Vitamin E:** Vitamin E is needed for normal stability of red blood cells. It has been shown to be essential for normal reproduction and for integrity of the muscles and nerves[109].

* **Arginine:** Arginine is an essential amino acid[110]. Its fundamental use is as a building block for body proteins such as enzymes, hormones, vitamins and structural proteins[111], and as a detoxifying agent[112]. Eighty percent of the male seminal fluid is made up of arginine.

* **Alanine:** This is an amino acid that is necessary for the synthesis of pantothenic acid[113].

* **Gamma Oryzanol**

* **Mexican Wild Yam Root**

* **Ginseng Root**

* **L-Alanine**

Memory Problems (Alzheimer's, Senility, Dementia)

Have you ever started to introduce friends or colleagues to one another but then could not recall their names? Have you ever looked at a phone number and, by the time you looked back at the phone to dial, you could not recall the last two or three digits? For some people these are everyday occurrences that make you feel very uncomfortable. However you can take heart, for these are "normal" situations according to the experts.

Even though the experts tell us that a little bit of forgetfulness is common, it does not help to alleviate the fear that something is wrong with you, and you may immediately jump to the conclusion that you have Alzheimer's disease.

The threat of Alzheimer's disease is enough to scare you into taking preventive action; if only you really knew what to do. In order to form a plan of action that would help protect you from this dreaded disease you need to understand exactly what causes it. Unfortunately, there is not much medical knowledge available. Why is this so?

There are many doctors who, by the very nature of their healing system, refuse to see diseases as the result of poor nutrition or caused by the American diet. It lies within a protective belief system because if they were to accept that the human body is the result of what goes into it, then they would have to accept that changing the input would change the results. This would also validate the health experts' claim that most diseases can be healed, controlled and/or prevented with good nutrition.

Those of us in the natural healing arts know that Alzheimer's is the result of poor nutrition and bad circulation. Let us first look at the circulation aspect. The blood is the lifeline of the body. It feeds each and every cell within the entire system. When it comes to the brain, it can only present the nutrients that the brain requires because blood does not enter into the brain matter.

There is a protective envelope surrounding the brain called the blood-brain barrier, and its purpose is to prevent blood from passing into the brain. The blood-brain barrier accepts the nutrients the brain needs and passes those through so the brain can feed and nourish itself. There are chemicals in the environment, the marketplace, in our food, air and water that may be able to transverse the blood/brain barrier.

If the blood is thick with cholesterol and triglycerides then the amount of nutrient-rich blood is severely restricted and the amount that passes by the barrier becomes even less. When this happens you can begin to imagine how little of the available nutrients are able to feed the brain, so it is no wonder that the brain is starving to death, dying a little bit each day. This may be the main reason that people begin to forget.

This brings us to the next area of concern, memory or your ability to recall information when you need it. The mind works because of neurotransmitters. Neurotransmitters are nutrients that act as "switches" in the brain. They allow the electrical nerve impulses to pass and permit all of the functions of the body to take place in proper sequence.

You can begin to imagine what can take place when the brain does not have an adequate amount of neurotransmitters, or nutrients, available to construct them. In electrical terms you would have a power failure, or a device would not work properly and may even burn up. The brain is confronted with the same kind of situation. It does not make the right or complete connections and, therefore, there is a "short." The mind goes blank or it begins to plug into an old, disconnected memory circuit.

We call this confusion, dementia, disorientation, memory lapse, senility or, of course, Alzheimer's disease. However, there is a way to fortify the brain with the proper nutrients to create neurotransmitters because neurotransmitters, like enzymes in the body, are the result of biochemical constructions.

Alzheimer's, senility, dementia and memory problems in general have different causes. I believe that they are fundamentally the result of malnutrition. There are many theories out there as to what causes Alzheimer's. One of the theories is that aluminum is in the brain, and once aluminum gets into the body it cannot be chelated out. However, modern science is undecided. If you think about it, many of us grew up eating out of aluminum cookware and glassware, such as the old spun aluminum glasses of the 1950s.

Another theory is based on findings of a protein plaque they have discovered in the brains of Alzheimer's patients.

One of the most important nutrients for the brain is oxygen; 25% of all the oxygen that you breathe goes to feed your brain. Oxygen is carried through hemoglobin to the blood-brain barrier. There the oxygen is passed into the brain environment and oxygen helps to nourish the brain along with other nutrients.

If we take into consideration that the number one killer in the country today is cardiovascular disease, primarily clogged arteries, then it is easy to see that there is not enough oxygen-rich blood flowing to the blood-brain barrier. The arteries are so constricted that not enough blood is reaching the barrier to pass oxygen to the brain. Consequently, it is my belief that Alzheimer's, senility and dementia are oxygen starvation problems.

Nutrients and Herbs for Memory

* **Choline:** Known as a fat burner and works to dissolve fats in the bloodstream.

* **Folic Acid:** Essential for mental and emotional health.

* **Inositol:** Co-functions with choline as a fat burner.

* **Lecithin:** Excellent fat metabolizer.

* **Magnesium:** Plays an important role in neuromuscular contractions.

* **Manganese:** Helps nourish the nerves and brain; aids in the utilization of choline.

* **Niacin/Niacinamide:** Improves circulation and reduces the cholesterol level in the blood.

* **Pantothenic acid:** Important for healthy skin and nerves and vital in cellular metabolism.

* **Potassium:** Unites with phosphorus to send oxygen to the brain. Also functions with calcium in the regulation of neuromuscular activity.

* **Selenium:** A natural antioxidant that appears to preserve elasticity of tissue by delaying oxidation of polyunsaturated fatty acids.

* **Unsaturated Fatty Acids:** Makes it easier for oxygen to be transported by the bloodstream. Helps perform a vital function in breaking up cholesterol deposited on arterial walls.

* **Vitamin B-1:** Has a beneficial effect on mental attitude and a healthy nervous system. It is linked with improved individual learning capability.

* **Vitamin B-6:** Promotes the normal functioning of the nervous and musculoskeletal systems.

* **Vitamin E:** Causes dilation of the blood vessels, permitting a fuller flow of blood.

* **Zinc:** May be involved in binding substances of vital function to the brain, as large deposits of zinc have been located in the brain.

* **L-Glutamine:** Readily crosses the blood-brain barrier in the brain where it is quickly converted into Glutamic acid. Serves primarily as a fuel for the brain, which also keeps excess amounts of ammonia from damaging the brain.

* **L-Methionine:** Helps nourish brain cells and supports choline's role in promoting thinking ability.

* **L-Taurine:** Both a neurotransmitter and mood elevator.

* **L-Tyrosine:** Stimulates production of norepinephrine, the "alertness" brain chemical. It plays a role in sharpening learning, memory and awareness, as well as elevating mood and motivation.

* **Acetylcholine:** The most important of the body's neurotransmitters (brain chemicals that carry messages between neurons, facilitate learning, memory and intelligence). Its key role is maximizing mental ability and prevents loss of memory in aging adults.

* **Glutamic Acid:** Principal amino acid contributes to brain-energy supplies.

* **Gotu Kola:** Specifically to improve memory and longevity. Excellent oxygen carrier.

* **PABA:** Allows electricity to jump from nerve ending to receptor sites.

* **Phosphatidyl Choline:** Acts as a fat metabolizer and is converted into acetylcholine, a neurotransmitter.

Menopause

In women, menopause seems to take place between forty to fifty years of age. It is believed that the main reason for the physical changes is that the ovaries are "burned out." The burnout occurs because the primordial follicles decrease with age and, as they decrease in number, the ability of the ovaries to produce estrogen also decreases.

Interestingly, not all women experience the same physical reactions as their bodies go through this particular transition. Some women experience virtually no affects at all. There are many different reasons for this variance. Lack of exercise, emotional stress and physical stress all can exaggerate the changes taking place. One of the most obvious influences is the nutritional status of the body, especially the adrenal glands.

Menopause is not a disease; it is a natural change within the female body when the body metabolically changes from being a potentially child bearing female to not.

Estrogen Production

Estrogen is primarily produced in the ovaries. The reduction of the primordial follicles or the removal of the ovaries can, therefore, account for the menopausal experience for women. However, there is another set of glands in the body that produces both the precursors for estrogen and progesterone; these are known as the adrenal glands. The health and vitality of the adrenals may be one reason why some women have an easier time with this natural transition.

Physical Effects of Menopause

The loss of estrogen often causes marked physiological changes in the function of the body. These changes include hot flashes, irritability, fatigue, anxiety and, occasionally, various mental/emotional states.

Nutritional Considerations

The first and foremost consideration in any normal transition within the body would be to nourish it so that it can maintain homeostasis, balance and harmony reflected as good health. If ovaries are present, nourish, rebuild, and re-stimulate estrogen production. If ovaries have been removed, then include natural herbs with estrogenic properties. In both instances nourish and fortify adrenal glands.

Nutrients and Herbs to Assist in Relieving Night Sweats and Hot Flashes:

* **Calcium:** Insufficient amounts cause a decrease in estrogen production. If there is not enough calcium in the blood for muscle use, it is "borrowed" from the bone[114]. According to the National Institute of Health, a healthy premenopausal woman should have about 1,000 to 1,200 mgs per day. The Institute further suggests that a post-menopausal woman consume 1,200 to 1,500 mgs per day to help avoid bone loss[115].

* **Pantothenic Acid:** Nourishes the adrenal glands. Also becomes Betaine HCL, which is essential for carrying the calcium ion into the bone matrix during the rebuilding process.

* **Vitamin B-6:** Excellent for women who are susceptible to finger/joint pain that often accompanies menopause.

* **Vitamin C:** Found in large quantities within the adrenal glands. It is also needed in sex glands as aging takes place.

* **Vitamin E:** An antioxidant that helps prevent oxidation of the hormones produced in the adrenal glands.

* **Dong Quai:** Considered one of the best herbs for females because it does many different things within the reproductive system.

*   **Iodine:** Nourishes the thyroid and is an essential trace element that is an integral part of the thyroid hormones, thyroxine and triiodothyronine. These hormones help to regulate metabolism and activity of the nervous system.

*   **Licorice Root and Wild Yam Root:** Have both been used to provide estrogen-mimicking properties to the body.

*   **Passion Flower:** Great for calming the nerves, much like a tranquilizer.

*   **Unicorn Root:** Cleanses and strengthens ovaries.

Menses (Irregular)

Irregular periods have myriad causes. More often than not, it is because the reproductive system is out of balance, usually caused by poor nutrition. For nutritional guidance refer to the section on Fertility and the nutrients there. That will help bring the system back into its normal cycle.

If there is cramping, that condition is usually the result of poor mineralization. See the section on Minerals for more information. When there is bloating, refer to the water balance section under Water Rentention.

Heavy bleeding and prolonged bleeding can be an indication of Vitamin K and mineral deficiency. Vitamin K, along with calcium, helps blood to clot. For Vitamin K, you want to consider taking a 100 microgram tablet two to three times for the first two days. As the bleeding stops, reduce or eliminate the Vitamin K.

Migraine

Despite the debates over causation, in the health food industry the only fundamental approach for migraines is the herb, Feverfew, along with Vitamin B-6, 100 mgs. I would take both three times a day. You could double up on the Feverfew.

Minerals

I am a firm believer in minerals. I feel that people do not get enough minerals in their foods or multiple vitamins. Even when you buy a calcium or a cal-mag or a cal-mag-zinc supplement, you are still denying yourself phosphorous, potassium, manganese, chromium and selenium. Minerals are essential, especially when dealing with leg aches, back aches, charley horses, restless leg syndrome, TMJ, growing pains, insomnia, palpitations, tossing and turning all night, and spasms. These are all indications that the body's mineral supply is compromised.

Minerals act as the major transmission junctions and switches for the electrical message impulses that flow from the brain to the muscles. These impulses use the nervous system as the transmission lines. The nervous system, like a "telephone" line, carries messages to and from the brain. The minerals are the switches that allow the electric impulses to flow without disruption or disturbance.

Minerals are engaged in almost every physical reaction in the body. You could not breathe, eat or drink without the aid of minerals. Minerals are absolutely essential for health.

Minerals necessary to maintain homeostasis:

Calcium	Manganese
Chromium	Phosphorus
Copper	Potassium
Iodine	Selenium
Iron	Zinc
Magnesium	

Calcium is a mineral that is necessary for healthy, strong bones and teeth. Other functions of the calcium ion include its influence in blood coagulation, neuromuscular excitability,

cellular adhesiveness, transmission of nerve impulses, maintenance and function of cell membranes, and activation of enzyme reactions and hormone secretion. When calcium levels in
the blood are abnormally low, hypocalcemia can occur. Some
symptoms of hypocalcemia are tetany, increased neuromuscular irritability, seizures and cardiac cramps. Low levels of calcium can also lead to reduced skeletal mass. Calcium absorption
is dependent on the amount of exposure a person has to ultraviolet light, vitamin D intake, the sex and age of the individual
and the bioavailability of calcium.

Chromium is involved in carbohydrate, lipid and nucleic
acid metabolism. It functions in carbohydrate and lipid metabolism as a potentiator of insulin action. In nucleic acid metabolism, it is postulated to be involved in maintaining the structural integrity of the nuclear strands and regulation of gene
expression. One of the first signs of a chromium deficiency is
glucose intolerance. Others include elevated circulating insulin,
glycosuria, fasting hyperglycemia, elevated serum cholesterol
and triglycerides, neuropathy and encephalopathy.

Copper is important in the formation of red blood cells
and bones. Copper is part of many enzymes and works with
Vitamin C to form elastin. Menkes syndrome, neutropenia,
which results in an increased susceptibility to infections, mi-
crocytic anemia, abnormal metabolism of carbohydrates and
impaired glucose tolerance are all symptoms of a deficiency of
this important mineral. Uncooked meat, high intakes of zinc,
iron, phosphorus and ascorbic acid are inhibitory factors to
the absorption and utilization of this nutrient.

Iodine is an essential part of the hormones thyroxine and
triiodothyronine. These hormones are required for normal
growth and development and for maintenance of a normal
metabolic state. Iodine is also needed for the prevention of
goiter. Deficiency symptoms include endemic goiter, endemic
cretinism, endemic deafmutism and endemic neuropsychic re-

tardation. Iodine's only function in the body is as a component of the thyroid hormones. There are no substances or outside events that will affect the body's ability to absorb and utilize this nutrient.

Iron is essential to vertebrate forms of life because its role in the heme molecule is central in permitting oxygen and electron transport. It is necessary for protein metabolism, immune system resistance, growth, healthy teeth, skin, nails and bones. It is also needed for the formation of hemoglobin and myoglobin. When the body is low on iron, iron deficiency anemia can result. Although it causes few deaths, it does contribute to the weakness, ill health and substandard performance of millions of people. Iron deficiency results from one or a combination of the following: impaired absorption, blood loss, or repeated pregnancies. Iron deficiency in adults is rarely due to an iron-poor diet alone. Excessive zinc and phosphorus can work against the absorption and utilization of this mineral.

Magnesium is essential for the normal metabolism of potassium and calcium. It is also required for the mobilization of calcium from bone. When it is absorbed and retained, it is used for tissue growth, which includes bone growth, and for turnover replacement. Magnesium plays a key role as an essential prosthetic group in at least 300 enzymatic reactions in intermediary metabolism. Magnesium deficiency symptoms include Trousseau's and Chvostek's signs, muscle fasciculation, tremor, muscle spasm, personality changes, anorexia, nausea and vomiting. There are no substances or outside events that will affect the body's ability to absorb and utilize this mineral.

Manganese promotes enzyme activation. High levels of this nutrient can be found in the bones, liver and pituitary gland. Manganese deficiency has never been reported in free-living humans. An excessive iron deficiency will lead to increased manganese absorption in humans. Therefore, iron deficiency could make an individual more vulnerable to manganese toxicity. At the same time, manganese over-exposure might induce anemia by blocking iron absorption.

Phosphorus plays fundamental roles in modifying the development and maturation of bone, in governing renal excretion of hydrogen ions and in modifying the effects of the B vitamins. Also, this mineral is essential for the metabolism of carbohydrate, fats and protein. Because it plays a role in bone resorption, mineralization and collagen synthesis, it plays an integral role in calcium homeostasis. Phosphate depletion syndromes in humans are often the result of inappropriate ingestion of non-absorbable antacids. However, the syndrome is readily reversed when the antacids are discontinued and sufficient amounts of dietary phosphate are consumed.

Potassium is stored almost entirely within the lean tissues, where it serves as the dominant intracellular cation. Potassium deficiency causes urinary ammonium wasting. Decreased total body potassium can lead to hypokalemia. This can cause impaired glucose tolerance with impaired insulin secretion, cardiac effects, impaired protein synthesis, respiratory and vocal cord muscle weakness.

Selenium preserves tissue elasticity and works with Vitamin E. Like vitamins A, C and E, selenium is an anti-oxidant.

Zinc aids in the digestion and metabolism of phosphorus and protein. It is a component of insulin and of male reproductive fluid. It is necessary for the healing processes involved with burns and wounds, and it is involved with prostate gland functions and carbohydrate digestion. Sterility, delayed sexual maturity, loss of taste, poor appetite, fatigue and retarded growth are all symptoms of a zinc deficiency.

Trace or Microminerals are needed in minute quantities. The best sources of microminerals are sea vegetables, such as kelp and algae.

Dietary suggestions:

* Avoid red meats. Animal protein contains phosphates that may compromise calcium absorption.

* Organically grown fruits and vegetables can be good sources of minerals without the added problems of pesticides and herbicides.

* Sea vegetables are good sources of minerals.

Lifestyle suggestions:

Avoid excessive stress. Exercise regularly. Weight bearing exercise is important to the maintenance of the skeletal structure. Astronauts have to perform special exercises during low- or no-gravity space travel to avoid loss of important minerals.

Miscarriage

Miscarriages may be the result of many different extenuating circumstances, especially poor nutrition. One of the end results, or contributing factors, would be weak uterine walls. As the fetus grows it cannot remain adhered to the wall, and thus there is a miscarriage. Nutrients essential for strengthening the uterine walls can be found in the female fertility nutrients. (See Fertility section).

Nails

Your nails can tell you a little about your health. If you have white specks on your nails, that is an indication that you need zinc. On the other hand, if your nails are wavy like a roller coaster, that tells me you have an issue with protein assimilation. Your diet may be heavy in protein, but you may not be assimilating it. In that case, look at digestive enzymes, look at your pancreas, and look at detoxifying your liver.

Brittle nails indicate a need for protein and minerals.

Nerve and Muscle Function

Each time you talk with someone in the healing arts, you are bound to get different perceptions of the same truth. However, there is one thing all healers agree upon, whether they are allopathic (commonly referred to as medical doctors), osteopaths, homeopaths, naturopaths or faith/psychic healers, and that is nerve transmission and proper muscle function is vital to good health.

Nerve Function

Without proper nerve transmissions, your body would die. The nerves act like telephone lines; they receive the messages from the brain and transmit them through nerve "lines" to their correct destinations. Each destination point then reacts in a very specific way based upon the directive of the message sent from the brain.

Muscles and Muscle Function

The muscles play an entirely different role than the nerves. Muscles are a kind of tissue made up of fibers that are able to expand and contract, allowing movement throughout the body.

The heart muscle (myocardium) is sometimes called a third (cardiac) kind of muscle. However, it is basically a striated muscle that does not contract as quickly as the skeletal muscles, and is not completely paralyzed if it loses stimulation.

Nutritional Needs

Minerals play an important role in the transmission of impulses between the nerves and the cells that make up muscles. Minerals are part of all body tissues and fluids, and are important factors in keeping physiological processes going. They act in nerve responses and muscle contractions, regulate electrolyte balance, the making of hormones, and become parts of enzymes.

Even if minerals are contained in the current multiple you are using, you know you need them when you have any of the following symptoms: shoulder, back or leg aches, cramps, spasms, palpitations, trouble falling asleep, or toss and turn all night long.

If you can relate to these symptoms, then you need minerals. Take them thirty minutes or so before going to bed. You will sleep soundly and wake up without feeling drugged.

Nutrients to Support the Nervous and Muscular Systems:

* **Calcium:** Calcium influences neuromuscular excitability and transmission of nerve impulses. When calcium levels in the blood are low, symptoms of increased neuromuscular irritability, seizures and cardiac cramps are possible.

* **Inositol:** Necessary for the metabolism of fats and cholesterol, and for the formation of lecithin.

* **Magnesium:** Deficiency symptoms include muscle fasciculation (involuntary twitching), tremors and muscle spasms.

* **Niacin:** Promotes growth and proper nervous system function. Deficiency symptoms include insomnia, tiredness and nervous disorders.

* **Vitamin B-6:** Necessary for the nerves, muscles and digestion. A deficiency will cause nervousness and irritability.

Obesity (See Weight Loss and Water Retention)

Osteoporosis

Osteoporosis affects both women and men, although women more frequently suffer from the condition. Aside from age-related hormonal changes, one major cause of osteoporosis is a diet rich in protein. Protein foods (meat, fish, foul, nuts, grains, etc.) leave an acid ash in the bloodstream, whereas fruits and vegetables leave an alkaline ash.

Ash is the residue of metabolic processes. Eating a diet high in protein and other acid-forming foods means that the calcium in the bloodstream will attempt to neutralize the acidity in order to maintain an alkaline state.

The body's innate intelligence seeks to keep a slightly greater alkaline level because germs, a catchall term, cannot survive in an alkaline environment. This is a self-protective measure, but to do so it uses available bloodstream calcium ions, thus forcing the body to pull from reserves, such as the bones or wherever else it can. This constant pulling of calcium from the bones contributes to the cause of osteoporosis.

Nutrients, Herbs and Digestive Enzymes to Support Bone Health:

*   **Calcium:** Magnesium, Phosphorus, and Zinc. Essential for calcium assimilation.

*   **Vitamin A:** Vital to any growth and development because bone is constantly changing and being remodeled.

*   **Vitamin C:** Essential to production of collagen, which is the substance that gives bone its flexibility.

*   **Vitamin D and Betaine Hydrochloride:** For calcium assimilation.

*   **Zinc:** Needed for the protein formation of bone.

*   **Alfalfa:** Contains easily-assimilated forms of calcium.

*   **Horsetail Grass:** For silica content.

*   **Phosphorus**

Palpitations

I always envision palpitations as being similar to electrical short circuits. Consider that muscle contractions, as well as relaxation, require calcium and magnesium for the electricity of thought to reach cells to communicate with them so they know what to do.

Cramping occurs when the muscles contract and stay contracted, and there is not enough magnesium to allow the electrical impulse of relaxation to reach the cells to allow the muscles to relax. In palpitation, it is like a flickering light—contact/no contact; contraction/relaxation. Without adequate magnesium, that back and forth situation occurs. Palpitations are best handled by working with a complete multi-mineral. (See Minerals).

Parasites

Parasites enter the body through different channels. It could be from the water a person drinks or from being in a river or lake that is parasite infested. Most parasites enter the body through the food we eat.

There are many different schools of thought in relation to parasites and the role they play in creating disease. A recent healer and author stated that parasites were a cause of diabetes. The theory is that they invade the pancreas, thereby interfering with its functioning. In this way, the insulin-producing capabilities of the pancreas are reduced and excessive sugar builds up in the bloodstream.

Another healer feels that parasites are the cause of tumors and cysts. Still others believe parasites in the intestinal tract rob the body of needed nutrients, thus lowering health and vitality, which sets in motion the receptivity for disease.

Regardless of what role or roles you believe parasites play in illness, it is still prudent to eliminate them from the body, and the easiest way to do it is with herbs.

The ideal way to take the herbs is in capsule form. Take them for four days and then stop for four days. This will give the eggs a chance to hatch. Then take the capsules again for another four days, then four days off.

Herbs to Assist the Body in Eliminating Parasites from the Intestinal Tract:

* **Black Walnut:** Used to expel various kinds of worms.

* **Butternut Root Bark:** Most mild and efficacious laxative known.

* **Garlic:** Increases resistance to bacterial infection and has been proven to have this effect on multiple germs. Combats the following fungi; Candida albicans, microsporum and epidermophyton.

* **Papaya Seeds:** Used extensively in Mexico as a way of ridding the body of parasites and worms.

* **Pau D'Arco:** Used in all situations that deal with bacteria.

* **Pumpkin Seeds:** High in zinc; employed to kill parasites.

* **Wormseed:** Also known as Jerusalem Artichoke. Known for its ability to kill parasites.

Premenstrual Syndrome

Premenstrual Syndrome (PMS) has generated a lot of interest over the past few years as medicine and nutritional science have debated whether to acknowledge the existence of this condition. In keeping with the philosophy of nutritional science that each disease or discomfort results from nutritional deficiencies, supplementation offers one of the more sensible approaches to countering the symptoms of PMS. The most commonly reported symptoms include fluid retention, bloating, painful breasts, headaches, backaches, skin eruptions, mental depression, irritability and lethargy.

Interestingly, many of these symptoms are the same for Candida, and some women have a discharge prior to their menstrual cycle. Is it possible that, as the body prepares to cleanse, it experiences a level of stress sufficient to lower the immune system, thus allowing the Candida to temporarily flourish?

Any change in the body's internal balance can create stress, and stress attacks the body by taxing the adrenal glands, which secrete hormone messengers that tell the other glands how to perform or what to manufacture. When the adrenal glands are taxed and begin to falter, so does the immune system. This is why when you are under stress everything seems to be worse, and what has been held at bay now can flourish. Conditions such as acne, allergies, Candida, herpes, shingles and hypoglycemia all flourish.

All the body's glands and systems are interconnected and interdependent. That is why a proper nutritional balance is so vital to attaining and maintaining health. A strong nutritional state also greatly reduces or eliminates the opportunity for disease to take hold.

Nutrients and Herbs to Prevent Common Symptoms Associated with PMS:

* **Calcium:** Acts as a calming agent and relieves backaches.

* **Iron:** Depletion can cause a variety of symptoms, including fatigue, inability to concentrate, paleness and lack of muscle tone.

* **Magnesium:** For the assimilation of calcium. Relaxes muscles and nerves.

* **Pantothenic Acid:** Nourishes the adrenal glands; helps to provide energy.

* **Vitamin B-1:** Known as the "morale vitamin" for its beneficial effect on the nervous system and mental attitude.

* **Vitamin B-6:** Helps maintain the balance of sodium and potassium, which regulates body fluids and promotes normal functioning of the nervous and musculoskeletal systems.

* **Vitamin C:** Along with zinc and vitamins B-6 and B-3 (niacin), this nutrient is a vital co-factor in the production of additional GLA (Gama Linolenic Acid).

* **Zinc:** Another co-factor for GLA.

* **Blessed Thistle:** For headaches and any kind of female problem.

* **Corn Silk:** Used extensively for the reduction of fluids.

* **False Unicorn Root:** Helps in reducing headaches and depression.

* **Horsetail Grass:** One of the best sources of silica that is essential for calcium assimilation and utilization. Silica also transmutes into calcium.

* **Licorice Root:** Estrogenic activity.

* **Parsley:** Excellent for reducing fluid retention.

* **Squaw Vine:** Good for morning sickness or nausea. Also contains significant amounts of the amino acid tryptophan, known for its calming effects.

* **Suma:** Invigorates the female hormonal balance without disturbing effects.

* **Valerian Root:** Valerian root and its major constituents, called valepotriates, have marked sedative, anticonvulsive, hypotensive, tranquilizing, neurotropic and anti-aggression properties.

* **Watermelon Seeds:** Good for reducing fluids.

* **Wild Lettuce:** Has a sedative effect on the central nervous system.

* **Phosphorus**

* **Potassium**

Prostate Problems

Located directly under the urinary bladder and surrounding the superior portion of the urethra from its origin in the bladder, the prostate is the largest accessory gland of the male reproductive tract, and is composed of muscular and glandular tissues.

The prostate slowly increases in size from birth to puberty, then grows at an increased pace, attaining a stable size during the third decade of life. It remains stable in size until about the age of forty-five, when further enlargement may occur. For reasons not yet completely understood, the prostate can frequently increase in size at an older age to a point that two out of three men reaching the age of seventy can suffer from some degree of urinary obstruction.

The Function of the Prostate

The function of the prostate is to secrete a milky, slightly acidic fluid into the prostatic urethra, through its many prostatic ducts. The urethra is the terminal canal for the male reproductive and urinary systems, and serves as a passageway for the different fluids that interact to form semen.

Prostatic fluid contains enzymes that balance the acid levels of the interacting fluids and help in the movement function of sperm, the male transporter of life. Prostatic fluid also tempers acid levels in sperm stored in the ductis deferens.

There is a good deal of research being conducted on the prostate, yet it remains one of the least understood structures in the body. One area of study concentrates on the major function of the gland, the production and the secretion of citrates. Citrates are part of the circular chain of cellular respiration, known as the Kreb's Cycle.

The Kreb's Cycle is the process in which a sequence of enzymatic reactions involving the metabolism of carbon chains of sugars, fatty acids and amino acids yields carbon dioxide, water and high-energy phosphate bonds. The Kreb's cycle provides a major source of adenosine triphosphate energy and produces molecules that are the starting point for a number of vital metabolic pathways, including amino acid synthesis. It also releases carbon dioxide from the cells for respiratory expulsion from the lungs.

Interestingly, correlations exist between citrate production and zinc accumulation in the human prostate. For example, it is known that the hormone testosterone stimulates zinc uptake and concentration in prostate, which parallels its stimulation of citrate accumulation and secretion[116].

Sperm

Sperm is acidic due to the metabolic end products, so the infusion of prostatic fluids into the ejaculatory duct serves to regulate the acidity of the sperm. Also, female vaginal secretions are acidic (with a pH of 3.5 to 4.0) and sperm do not become optimally motile until the pH of the surrounding fluids rises anywhere from 6 to 6.5.

Prostatic fluids in the sperm neutralize the acidity after ejaculation, which would enhance the sperm's motility and fertility.

Many men over the age of fifty seem to suffer from an inflamed prostate gland. The inflammation is sometimes painful and almost always uncomfortable. By eliminating the physical causes, you may be able to increase the speed of healing. Another step would be to increase the use of those nutrients that are known to be beneficial to the prostate.

Nutrients, Amino Acids and Herbs for Prostate Support:

*   **Magnesium:** As a component of calcium homeostasis, magnesium works in the prostate to help with the utilization of calcium.

* **Vitamin E and Unsaturated Fatty Acids:** Essential for glandular health; they work together in the lessening of residual urine. Vitamin E plays a role in prostate support by protecting the fat-soluble vitamins; vitamin A, with its role in epithelial cells; and vitamin D, essential for maintaining prostate health.

* **Zinc:** An essential mineral for normal prostate gland function. A component of semen; it is believed that at least 1 mg of zinc is excreted in one ejaculem. There are also major losses of zinc in the intestinal tract. Physiological functions of zinc include fertility, reproduction and sexual maturity.

* **Alanine:** Glutamic Acid, Glycine. Vital amino acids are important; their role in human nutrition is extensive and not fully known.

* **Bee Pollen:** Contains various nutrients that strengthen and benefit the body.

* **Gravel Root and Parsley:** Herbs used traditionally for their inflammation reducing properties.

* **Pumpkin Seeds:** High in zinc.

* **Glutamic Acid**

* **L-Glycine**

Psoriasis

I have always perceived psoriasis as a kind of an invasion of the skin by the trillions of little microbes that live on it. Psychic trauma creates a hospitable environment for them to burrow into the skin.

Your skin has what is called an acid mantle. This literally protects you from microbial invasion. However, when there is trauma of such deep nature that the body momentarily loses its integrity due to the shock, the immune system is diminished.

At that moment the microbes have an opportunity to burrow into the skin. With that belief in mind, I use peppermint oil and lemongrass oil to kill the microbes.

Here is a formula to make your own ointment: Make an oil to apply topically using the essential oils of lemongrass and peppermint. Add one part each of lemongrass and peppermint oils to six parts almond oil.

Restless Leg Syndrome

This is another issue regarding minerals. Just like cramps and palpitations, it is a matter of calcium and magnesium not being present in adequate amounts. The minerals could be depleted for so many different reasons—stress, a high protein diet, and/ or a lack of sufficient amounts of vegetables coming into the system (which provide natural calcium). Dairy is not necessarily the best source of calcium.

For all of these reasons, there is a breakdown in electrical communication within the body. So, restless leg, palpitations, charley horses and cramps all fall under the same category of not having enough minerals in the system to accomplish all of the transactions for which minerals are essential. (See Minerals).

Shingles (See Herpes)

Sinus Infections

Sinus infections are often in fact fungal infections. Although the fungal infections could have sources other than Candida, the sinus infections (thrush, ear infections) are generally Candida overgrowth—Candida infections.

Candida is natural to the throat; but, again, here is an issue of stress taxing the adrenals and the adrenals faltering, then the bacteria having a chance to flourish, grow and spread.

You could use the nasal douche approach and work with a neti pot. If you choose to do that, you will want to use the herbs goldenseal root or Oregon sea grape, pau d'arco and black walnut. Be sure to use goldenseal root or Oregon sea grape as they both contain berbine, the active anti-fungal and mold eliminator. Make a strong pot of tea and use as a nasal douche.

To make the nasal douche tea: Bring to boil 8 ounces of distilled water. Remove from heat. Add 1 tablespoon of each herb. Strain and use the tea when it is at room temperature. You may want to throw in a pinch of clean salt.

Skin Issues

Skin issues manifest in many forms – from acne (covered earlier), to other kinds of strange growths or outcroppings on the skin. Most issues with the skin, like warts, will end up being of a viral or fungal bacteria origin. I believe as well that they play a part in psoriasis.

Toxins can also play a role in issues with the skin, because your skin is the largest eliminative organ of the body. When your body is ridding itself of toxic material/poisons from within, they deposit on the skin and the billions of microbes that live on our skin interact with the toxins. As a result, eruptions and other manifestations will appear.

Vitamin A, zinc, niacin and selenium are all excellent for the skin. However, when you are dealing with something topical, whatever is on your skin needs to be approached from that angle – topically.

In that regard, you want to make an oil to apply topically using the essential oils of lemongrass and peppermint. Add one part each of lemongrass and peppermint oils to six parts almond oil. The body will absorb it very quickly. Apply it wherever you have warts or anything on your skin that you are not sure of.

Vitiligo is a pigmentation loss, but I would also use these two oils and a wash made out of goldenseal root, pau d' arco, myrrh and black walnut. To make the wash, bring eight ounces of distilled water to a boil. Remove from heat and add to water one tablespoon of each herb. Then strain the herbs from the mixture and use frequently. All of these herbs are antibiotic in nature.

You could also take some organic cornmeal and make a paste out of that, or a mush, and cover your affected parts. In South America, it is one of the methods used for eliminating foot fungus amongst the workers who are clearing the Amazon forest.

Spasms (See Minerals)

Stress, Tension and Hyperactivity

It is often said that stress is a killer, both directly and indirectly. Too much stress is known to be one cause of heart attacks, high blood pressure, strokes and depression. It contributes to lowered adrenal function and a depressed immune system. Stress creates physical tension.

Tension is when the muscles contract and fail to relax. When there is tension in the muscles, this limits the amount of blood that can flow through the arteries, veins and capillaries located in that area. When blood flow is reduced due to tension, pain or cramping can occur in that area. Heart attacks are an example of what happens when blood is reduced to an area. It is also true that elevated cholesterol levels can lead to heart attacks.

Another good example of stress and tension at work is the common headache. These are usually brought on by stress, and once the muscles tense and blood flow is reduced the headache begins. Blood carries oxygen and other nutrients to nerves and muscles, especially the brain, and when it becomes starved you begin to experience pain. Oxygen starvation can lead to diminished mental capacity.

The environment causes some forms of stress. This includes the air we breathe, water we drink, food we eat and places we work. Because of all these different sources of stress, both mental and physiological, it is important to maintain an excellent diet and fortify the body with those nutrients that will help the body deal with stress.

A healthy and nutritionally sound body deals with the stresses of life from a position of strength. This means that although there is stress from many different areas in your life, the body is not adversely affected by it.

Stress lowers the immune system by adversely affecting the adrenal glands, which subsequently can allow many conditions and diseases to flourish.

Unfortunately, the American diet does not contain enough nutrients to keep the body fit and able. Stress depletes nutrients such as calcium, vitamin C and the entire range of B-complex vitamins, and this depletion can cause feelings of nervousness, irritability, sleeplessness, muscle cramping and other physical ailments. The best way to deal with these depletions is to provide the body with the nutrients necessary.

Hyperactivity is often the result of stimulating chemicals brought into the body via the diet. The body is over-stimulated and, when the mineral content of the body is too low, hyperactivity manifests. The minerals act to maintain balance and harmony between the contraction and relaxation of the muscles and nerves.

Nutrients, Amino Acids and Herbs to Nourish and Relax Nerves:

* **B-complex Vitamins:** Work together in the nervous system and are involved in energy production and fat and protein metabolism.

* **Calcium and Magnesium:** Work to nourish and relax nerves and muscles. Calcium is the dominant mineral that is lost to stress. The loss of calcium disrupts the relation-

ship between sodium and potassium, potentially causing an individual to retain water and immediately gain five to fifteen pounds.

* **Inositol:** Helps calm the nervous system.

* **Vitamin B-6:** Essential for healthy nerve endings.

* **L-Tyrosine:** An amino acid known to elevate moods.

* **Hops, Skullcap and Valerian Root:** All used for ages to nourish, soothe and relax the nerves and muscles.

* **Niacinamide**

Throat Infections

A throat infection could be caused by Candida, as we discussed above in Sinus Infections, or it could be a germ or viral infection.

To alleviate the discomfort of a throat infection, you can mash garlic in honey and let it slowly coat the sore area. The garlic, as an irritant, will draw fresh antibodies more quickly to stop the infection and help remove debris caused by the infection.

Another healing approach is through fortifying the immune system. Here are the ideal immune system support nutrients:

* **Vitamin A:** A fat-soluble nutrient that plays an important role in the immune system and the healthy formation of mucous membranes, part of the body's outer protection against foreign toxins. The membranes release mucus in the linings of the mouth and nose, the digestive tube and the breathing passages. Mucus is composed of water, cast off tissue cells, mucin and white blood cells—the leukocytes. Leukocytes function as the catalyst for the B-cells and T-cells in the immune response process.

* **Vitamin C** has many uses in the body. It is essential for the immune system, playing a role in the absorption of iron and in the production of collagen.

* **Garlic, Reishi Mushroom, Elderberry, Goldenseal Root and Myrrh:** These are all known to be great antibiotics.

Thrush

Thrush is a Candida overgrowth that one can experience, especially when there is a high degree of stress. Even though the general cause is stress, infants get it more than adults. You would not think that babies and children have stress, yet research and diseases demonstrate otherwise.

Thrush can be treated the same as Laryngitis and Throat Infections. If there is an infection causing it, use the same kind of solution – the honey, garlic, vitamins A and C, and zinc (a zinc lozenge would be wonderful).

For babies, use the same tea for Candida infections, administered through bottle feeding. Immediately after the thrush is cleared, introduce probiotics as quickly as possible. This is important. Goldenseal root and Oregon sea grape contain a chemical the berbine, which attacks friendly intestinal bacteria, which have to be replaced.

Thymus Concerns

The thymus gland is a key component of the immune system. It is here that the T-cells called phagocytes, a variety of white blood cell, mature. These cells are constantly patrolling, seeking out and destroying pathogens and cells that do not belong in the body. There are different types of T-cells that help keep the body safe from invasion and disease.

Your immune system is your first line of defense against many of today's diseases, including cancer. Sickness begins at the cellular level, involving one or more cells. The path toward disease starts with the diet and then progresses. When the cells do not have a chance to mature into T-cells, there is no control over cell-mediated responses. To be on the safe side, especially with the threat of cancer, AIDS and other diseases in the world, it may pay to ensure that this gland stays in top shape.

Nutrients and Amino Acids to Support the Thymus Gland:

* **Beta-carotene (Vitamin A):** Converted into a non-toxic form of vitamin A in the body. Feeds and strengthens the thymus gland, which is instrumental in the body's response to infection.

* **Lecithin:** Increases resistance to diseases by helping the thymus gland carry out its functions.

* **Zinc:** Protects the immune system and supports the T-cells

* **L-Arginine:** A growth hormone that acts on the thymus gland to improve its ability to process T-effectors and B-cell lymphocytes.

* **L-Glycine:** Necessary for the immune system, balanced growth of white blood cells, and health of the thymus gland, spleen and bone marrow.

Thyroid Problems

Often called the "master gland" or "power control center," the thyroid is vital because of its interactions with other glands. It is also involved in sexual development and maturity. Goiters often result from low iodine content within the thyroid, which fills with blood.

The thyroid gland is located in the neck, just below the larynx (voice box). The thyroid gland is slightly heavier in women than in men, and becomes larger during pregnancy. The thyroid manufactures the hormones thyroxine and calcitonin.

The thyroid secretes these two hormones to influence the rate and processes of basic body metabolism and physical growth. There are two types of metabolism: catabolic and anabolic.

In catabolic metabolism, the body is in the process of breaking down tissues, cells and substances. These substances are simplified in their structure to speed up elimination and release energy.

In anabolic metabolism, the exact opposite process is taking pace. New material is being created, and nutrients are drawn from the blood into the cells to repair and grow new cells. The chemicals in the blood are used in the process of converting chemicals into parts of living cells.

The thyroid gland releases the hormone, thyroxine, directly into the blood after it is produced and secreted by the follicular cells. The hormone calcitonin is essential in the body because it influences calcium homeostasis. These two hormones require the nutrient iodine, a trace mineral, for production.

These thyroid hormones release a metabolic bi-product, triiodothyronine.

In cases of thyroid imbalance, the thyroid becomes either sluggish or overactive. When sluggish, the body retains fluids, adds weight and disrupts the natural flow of a woman's cycle. In the overactive mode, it creates nervousness and tension. It also causes inability to gain weight because the metabolism becomes so high that the body burns up everything that it takes in and the nerve cells work overtime until they become taxed, which can affect homeostasis.

Nutritional Support

The thyroid, like every other gland, organ or particular system of the body, requires very specific nutrients in order to function properly. The thyroid absolutely needs iodine for its nutritional support.

* **Chromium:** Can stimulate thyroid activity to initiate the mobilization of fat reserves for energy production.

* **Iodine:** Essential for the manufacturing of thyroxin, a thyroid hormone that helps influence and regulate metabolism.

* **Manganese:** Essential for the formation of thyroxin.

* **Vitamin B-6:** Excellent at metabolizing fats, proteins and carbohydrates.

* **Tyrosine:** Plays an integral role in proper functioning of the adrenal, pituitary and thyroid gland.

* **Bladderwrack:** Used effectively for thyroid problems.

* **Kelp:** Contains iodine, in addition to other substances.

* **Irish Moss:** A form of kelp that provides iodine.

Tinnitus

Tinnitus, also known as ringing in the ears, may be due to poor circulation. My basic approach to this is to clean out the arterial system, the carotid arteries, so that you can deliver more blood to the head and scalp, thus feeding the area around the ears.

You can try the traditional Mexican healer approach. Take a garlic clove, put a thread through it and place it in the ear. Let the clove stay there for an hour or so, then remove it with the thread. Do that two to three times a day.

A faster approach, and easier to apply, is to take a garlic pearl, puncture it and squeeze the garlic oil into the ear. Garlic, being an irritant, will draw blood to the area (same as with ear infections).

Tranquilizers

The ideal natural tranquilizers are minerals and certain herbs. (See the Nerve and Muscle Function nutrients and minerals). These groupings of minerals and herbs are ideal for inducing a tranquil state, relaxing the body and mind, and helping with anxiety.

* **Calcium** is a mineral necessary for healthy, strong bones and teeth. Other functions of the calcium ion include its

influence in neuromuscular excitability, cellular, and transmission of nerve impulses.

* **Magnesium** is essential for the normal metabolism of potassium and calcium.

* **Vitamin B-6** is necessary for the nerves and muscles, and digestion.

* **Valerian Root, Scullcap, Hops and Passion Flower** are all known to be excellent nervines, tranquilizers.

* **L-Tyrosine**

Ulcers

The most common types of ulcers are on the inside of the cheeks. This tells you there is too much protein in the diet.

Stomach ulcers are the next most common types of ulcers and can occur within the stomach lining or in the duodenum, the first part of the small intestines. Ulcers can also affect the intestinal tract. When this happens, the colon is usually the first site where they manifest, generally as ulcerative colitis. However, any segment of the intestinal tract can become ulcerated.

Ulcers can result from excess acid in your system. There is also a particular type of bacteria found in stomach ulcer sites, which is believed to create the ulcers.

In either case, stress seems likely to play a part in the process. In fact, there is a particular type of internal ulcer called a stress ulcer, which is seen primarily in post-surgical or burn patients. When we look at stress we see that it affects many different functions within the body and depletes nutrients.

Within the body, the adrenal glands are among those most directly impacted by stress. Stress diminishes their capacity to function, which can result in a less effective immune system. While in most instances the immune system will hold things in check, when stress becomes too intense, bacteria and other latent or opportunistic conditions can become active. Ulcers, either from direct stress or lowered immune function, will flourish.

The herbalist Dr. John Christopher prescribed a remedy for internal ulcers: mix one teaspoon of cayenne powder into a cup of hot water; let it stand to room temperature and drink immediately before going to bed. By the next morning the ulcer should be gone. I have heard that it works quite well. This treatment can last for years. Of course, if the original cause of the ulcer is not removed through understanding and control, there is a great likelihood that an ulcer will reappear.

Two other approaches, not as "tasty" as the first, are to drink one ounce of aloe vera juice as often as possible, or drink freshly made cabbage juice as often as possible. Keep in mind the potential for intestinal gases.

There are two other types of ulcers that a person can develop, however these are on the outside of the body: the diabetic ulcer, which is usually found around the ankles or on the feet; and bedsores, which usually develop in the skin over boney prominences in people who are bedridden or immobile.

Both of these types can be handled in the same fashion. Pour granulated sugar or raw honey into the ulcer. Either of these substances literally feeds the cells topically, and they create new, fresh skin. For bedsores, mix the sugar or honey with cornstarch and make a paste. Hospital employees have told me that some hospitals apply this strategy along with mixing sugar and iodine and smearing it across new incisions in the operating room.

Foods and Herbs to Assist the Body with Ulcers:

*   **Cabbage Juice:** A natural antiseptic used to ease ulcer pain; heals ulcers.

*   **Licorice Root:** Relieves ulcer conditions, also used for flavor.

*   **Marshmallow Root:** Soothes mucous membranes. Internally used to treat inflammation and mucosal afflictions of the genito-urinary tract.

* **Okra:** A very old, traditional approach to healing ulcers. It may stem from the mucilage nature of the vegetable.

* **Slippery Elm Bark:** Internally soothes irritated mucous membranes; valuable for mucous inflammation of the stomach. It will relieve ulcerated and cancerous stomachs.

Vaginitis

Vaginitis could be the result of a yeast infection, such as Candida or other bacteria. Use a strong herbal douche of all of the anti-fungal, anti-myocardial, anti-bacterial and anti-viral herbs, all mixed together. Use herbs like pau d'arco, black walnut, myrrh and goldenseal root. These are all extremely powerful in killing infections.

To make the tea:

1. Bring to boil 12 to 16 ounces of distilled water.

2. Remove from heat.

3. Add 2 tablespoons of each herb.

4. Let steep. Strain at room temperature.

5. Use as a douche.

Varicose Veins

Varicose veins are the same as hemorrhoids. They are distended veins. In hemorrhoids, it is due to pushing too hard and thus forcing the vein past its point of station. Varicose veins are usually the result of weak walls.

There are a couple of things you can do with varicose veins. One is the herb horse chestnut, taken in capsule form. Topically, you can approach varicose veins the same way you would a hemorrhoid, which is to make a poultice or oil out of white oak bark, bayberry bark and witch hazel (all of these are astringents). By applying the poultice topically, you will reduce the inflammation.

How to Make Oil for Varicose Veins:

1. Take a tablespoon each:
   * bayberry bark
   * white oak bark
   * slippery elm
   * witch hazel

2. Add about six ounces of olive oil.

3. Set in the sun for three days and let the sun cook the oil.

4. After three days, strain it and apply.

You can also add Super-C Complex to your mix: Vitamin C, bioflavonoids, rutin and hesperidin. I would do this on a daily basis, somewhere between 3000 mgs of vitamin C, 1500 mgs of the bioflavonoids, and 100 mgs of rutin. These nutrients will help strengthen the vascular walls and essentially eliminate bruising. By strengthening the capillaries and vascular walls, you will eliminate the further development of varicose veins.

Vision

The body's senses enable persons to observe what is taking place in the world around them and pass that vital information along to the brain and organs, whose health depends upon coping with the environment. The senses of touch, taste, sight, smell and sound play vital roles in our ability to adapt and thrive in the ever changing world.

For example, the sense of touch permits us to avoid serious injuries by sending sufficient messages to enable us to avoid extreme temperatures and textures. The shuddering you experience when you are exposed to a freezing rain or the quick muscle reaction you experience when touching a hot stove are simple examples of the manner in which the senses protect the human body.

Eyesight

Eyesight contributes to the overall health and well-being of the body. It is one of the five basic sensory tools people have to guide them through the world. Of course, eyesight has its limitations. We all know that good vision is never guaranteed freedom from harm, and accidents happen every day.

The eyes are amazing instruments. In some aspects, the eyes act much like cameras. Muscle contractions control both the focusing of the eyes and the filtering of light. The pupils react to light by expanding and contracting, maintaining the proper exposure for the retina.

The retina focuses on images in an inverted fashion; that is, the images are upside down and then reversed by the brain. An object that appears in the lower right-hand corner of the retina's frame of vision is actually in the upper left-hand corner of the field of vision. Early in life, the brain learns to coordinate the images, giving us a true picture of objects. The brain stores memories and automatically turns visual images right side up and right-side around[117].

The eyes communicate with the brain through the optic nerve. There are actually three systems involved in the function. The first system processes information related to the shape of the object, another system regards the color, and the third system handles information about movement, location and spatial organization of an image. Together the systems bring the image into focus and the brain reacts to whatever action the image requires.

Nutritional Support

The following information is provided to help you better understand the role that certain nutrients play in the nourishment of the eyes and the overall health of the body. Those nutrients are:

* **Vitamin A** contributes to the health of nearly every tissue in the body, and its role in vision is well understood. A modified light-receptive form of vitamin A, known as 11-cis-retinol, allows a person to see in very low light[118].

* **Vitamin E:** with its antioxidant properties, produces benefits in maintaining eye health.

* **B Comlplex** nutrients are required for the maintenance of ocular tissue and, in particular, the cornea and optic nerve.

* **Niacin** is necessary for growth, the proper functioning of the nervous system, and the transmission of impulses to the body's senses.

Other nutrients, while not directly associated with ocular health, contribute to the overall health of the body. This, in turn, may affect the health and well-being of the sensory functions.

Some of these nutrients include:

* **Vitamin D** is very important because it participates in healthy bone structure and muscular development.

* **Vitamin C** has many uses in the body. It increases the absorption of iron, helps in the production of collagen, and is essential for the immune system. Vitamin C is needed for healthy teeth, gums and bones while strengthening the blood vessels.

* **Calcium** is a mineral that is necessary for healthy, strong bones and teeth. Other functions of the calcium ion include its influence in blood coagulation, neuromuscular excitability and transmission of nerve impulses.

* **Magnesium** is essential for the metabolism of potassium and calcium.

* **Selenium** preserves tissue elasticity and works with Vitamin E. Like vitamins A, C and E, it is an antioxidant.

* **Zinc** aids in the digestion and metabolism of phosphorus and protein. Protein is essential for the forming of antibodies, enzymes and hormones.

Warts and Moles

A change in the appearance of a wart or mole is a sign of trouble. Warts are little viral enclaves on the body, where a virus has taken up residence and rooted itself, seeking to penetrate into the system. A mole is a birthmark, giving indication of sensitivity in a particular area.

Here is a formula to make your own ointment.

* Make an oil to apply topically using the essential oils of lemongrass and peppermint.

* Add one part each of lemongrass and peppermint oils to six parts almond.

Water Retention

Water retention, or edema, is a serious health problem. It directly contributes to obesity through the weight that is gained from water. Water retention can result from several things, however it generally stems from an imbalance in the potassium-sodium relationship.

Stress can easily disturb this balance because it depletes nutrients and calcium, in this case, at an accelerated rate. If those nutrients are not replaced in meaningful amounts, problems can arise. When calcium is depleted, the potassium-sodium ratio is disturbed, causing water to be retained.

Water retention can be a life and death issue, and as bad as high blood sugar. Excess water in the system puts pressure on the arterial system, thus elevating blood pressure, which could lead to a stroke and other issues.

The first amount of weight anyone loses is water; it is also the first thing that is retained when there is stress.

Nutrients and Herbs to Achieve Water Balance:

* **Potassium and Vitamin B-6:** Work together to maintain the fluid balance within.

* **Buchu Leaf, Corn Silk, Hydrangea, Parsley, Uva Ursi and Watermelon Seeds:** All excellent diuretics.

Weight Loss (See also Obesity)

Weight loss is a major topic unto itself with many ways to approach it. There are psychological concerns, as well as physiological, glandular effects at work in most everyone with weight issues.

Levels of stress affect weight, as well. Stress depletes calcium, which disrupts the relationship between potassium and sodium; and five to fifteen pounds can be gained immediately through water retention.

Successful weight loss requires true desire and commitment to the goal. This leads to discipline, which leads to success. The most difficult aspect of weight loss is changing the diet, due primarily to the myriad of emotional attachments and associations we all have with foods.

Some things are hard to give up, even when we know they are detrimental to our health.

Supplementation as Part of a Weight-Loss Program

In terms of incorporating natural supplements into weight-loss regimens, one has to be careful. There are many products offered, some of which can have negative effects. For instance, Guarana and other CNS (central nervous system) stimulators over-stimulate the nervous system. Personally I feel this is an unhealthy approach.

Traditionally, three safe and somewhat basic approaches have been used: (1) Diuretic-type herbs to reduce water content; (2) Lipo-tropic vitamins, better known as "fat burners," to reduce fat and cholesterol levels in the blood as well as fat/cholesterol "deposits" against the walls of the arteries; and (3) Natural appetite suppressants to curb the craving for food.

These approaches are effective and each works well in its own right. They are great complements to a healthy diet and exercise program, which will all work together to help you get control of your weight and to maintain control.

Nutrients, Amino Acids, and Herbs for Weight-Loss Programs

The following will support your body in burning fat, increasing basal metabolism, and flushing excess fluids from the body:

* **Choline, Inositol, and Lecithin:** These factors are used to reduce the fatty deposits within. Lecithin acts as a carrier of fat and it is urinated out of the body.

* **Iodine:** Essential for the manufacturing of thyroxin, a thyroid hormone that helps influence and regulate metabolism.

* **Potassium:** Acts as a diuretic by balancing fluids.

* **Vitamin B-6:** Acts as a diuretic.

* **L-Methionine:** An amino acid that aids the body in producing choline.

* **Kelp:** Contains iodine, which nourishes the thyroid gland and helps to regulate metabolism.

Epilogue

If you want to go further in the sense of understanding the emotional causes of diseases and conditions, take a look at my book *The Disease Symbology Handbook*, as well as my book, *The Dream Symbology Dictionary*. You may find both of them helpful in understanding the emotional conflicts that cause diseases and conditions.

I wish you the best of everything. Good health can be yours. Look at your diet and exercise, and practice positive thinking.

God Bless. Be well.

References

References

1. Gerald J. Tortora and Sandra Reynolds Grabowski, Principles of Anatomy and Physiology, 7th ed. (New York: HarperCollins, 1993), 91.

2. Federal Register, vol. 56, no. 229. Nov. 27, 1991, 60626.

3.Carol Jean West Suitor, M.S., R.D. and Merrily Forbes Crowley, R.N., M.S. Nutrition - Principles and Applications in Health Promotion, 2nd ed. (Philadelphia: J.B. Lippincott Co., 1984), 254.

4. Tortora and Grabowski, 91.

5. Federal Register, vol. 56, no. 229. Nov. 27, 1991, 60626.

6. Suitor and Crowley, 255.

7. Maurice E. Shils, M.D., Sc.D., and Vernon R.Young, Ph.D. Modern Nutrition in Health and Disease, 7th ed. (Philadelphia: Lea & Febiger, 1988), 343.

8. Suitor and Crowley, 255.

9. In China, centuries ago, the patient paid the doctor to stay well. So, the doctor treated them with herbs, such as the aforementioned, as a way of building the immune system to keep them healthy; because when they got sick, they had to be treated for free.

10. Tortora and Grabowski, 91.

11. Tortora and Grabowski, 601.

12. Tortora and Grabowski, 601.

13. Federal Register, vol. 56, no. 229. Nov. 27, 1991, 60627.

14. Suitor and Crowley, 255.

15. Federal Register, vol. 56, no. 229. Nov. 27, 1991, 60627.

16. Federal Register, vol. 56, no. 229. Nov. 27, 1991, 60625.

17. Shils and Young, 342, 344, 365

18. Suitor and Crowley, 254.

19. Suitor and Crowley, 254.

20. Schauss AG, et al. Journal of Agricultural and Food Chemistry 2006 Nov 1; 54(22):8604-10.

21. H.B. Allen, et al, "Oral Vitamin A in Acne Vulgaris," International Journal of Dermatology, 20(4) (1981): 278.

22.M. About-Khair, S. Fathi, M. Wahid, "Zinc in Human Health and Disease," Ric. Cl. Lab. 18 (1988): 0-16.

23. Judi Davis and Kim Sherer, Applied Nutrition and Diet Therapy for Nurses, 163, 573, 577.

24. Corinne H. Robinson, et al, Normal and Therapeutic Nutrition, 403-404, 523.

25. Robinson, et al, 403, 404, 523.

26. Kathleen L. Mahan and Sylvia Escott-Stump, Krause's Food, Nutrition and Diet Therapy, 143, 144, 890-894.

27. Sue Rodwell Williams, Nutrition and Diet Therapy, 961, 672, 959.

28. Williams, 961, 672, 959.

29. Davis and Sherer, 163, 573, 577.

30. C.H. Smith and W.R. Bidlack, "Dietary Concerns Associated with the Use of Medications," Journal of the American Dietary Association, 84(8) (1984): 901-14.

31. Tortora and Grabowski, 9.

32. Grace Burtis, Judi Davis, Sandra Martin, Applied Nutrition and Diet Therapy, (W.B. Saunders, 1987), 617.

33. Williams, 961, 672, 959.

34. Mahan and Stump, 143, 144, 890-894.

35. Mahan and Stump, 143, 144, 890-894.

36. A.J. Bollet, (1988) "Nutrition and diet in rheumatic diseases," In: Modern Nutrition in Health and Disease (Shils, M.E. & Young, V.N., eds.), (Lea and Febiger, Philadelphia, PA), 1362–1372.

37. Davis and Sherer, 163, 573, 577.

38. Melvyn R Werbach,, M.D. Nutritional Influences on IIlness, 328.

39. Bollet,1362–1372.

40. Bollet,1362–1372.

41. Mahan and Stump, 143, 144, 890-894.

42. "Recommended Dietary Allowance," National Academy of Science, 10th ed., (1989): 144.

43.Leon M. Chaitow, D.O., N.D., Amino Acids In Therapy, (Rochester, VT, 1985), 48.

44. Bollet,1362–1372.

45. Bollet,1362–1372.

46. Suitor and Crowley, 43, 46, 48, 49, 50, 262, 263.

47. Leonard Mervyn, B.SC., PhD., C. Chem., FRSC. Dictionary of Vitamins: Complete Guide to Vitamins and Vitamin Therapy, Member of New York Academy of Sciences, (Thorsons, 1984), 24, 58.

48. Suitor and Crowley, 43, 46, 48, 49, 50, 262, 263.

49. Suitor and Crowley, 43, 46, 48, 49, 50, 262, 263.

50. Sue Rodwell Williams, Nutrition and Diet Therapy (7th Ed.), (St. Louis: Mosby Publishing, 1990), 253.

51. Sherry A. Rogers, M.D., Tired or Toxic: A Blueprint for Health, (Syracuse NY: Prestige Publishing, 1990), 160.

52. Taber's Cyclopedic Medical Dictionary

53. Shekelle, R., Lepper, M., Liu, S., Maliza, C., Raynor, W.J., Rossof, A.H. (1981;ii:1985). Dietary vitamin A and risk of cancer in the western electric study. Lancet.

54. Kvale, G., Bjelke, E., Gart, J.J. (1983). Dietary habits and lung cancer risk. International of Journal Cancer, 31, 397.

55. Matthews-Roth, M.M. (1982). Antitumor activity of beta carotene, canthxanthin, and phytoene. Oncology, 39, 33.

56. Gouveia, J., Mathe, G., Hercend, T., Gros, F., Lemaigre, G., San-telli, G., et al. (1982). Degree of bronchial metaplasia in heavy smok-ers and its regression after treatment with a retinoid. Lancet, i, 710.

57. Goodman, D.S. (1984). Vitamin A and retinoids in health and disease. New England Journal of Medicine, 310(16), 1023.

58. Felter, HW The Eclectic Materia, Pharmacologhy and Thera-peutics Eclectic Medical Publications, Portland, OR, 1983 (first pub-lished in 1922.)

59. March 1985

60. Jan. 5th, 1978

61. Science News' Oct. 13th, 1984

62. Healing Nutrients Within Keats, 1987

63. Recommended Dietary Allowances (RDA), 169.

64. Victor Herbert and K.C. Das, "Folic Acid and Vitamin B12," in Modern Nutrition In Health and Disease, 9th ed., ed. M.E. Shils, et al, (Philadelphia: Williams & Wilkins, 1999), 404, 405.

65. The Bantam Medical Dictionary.

66. The Bantam Medical Dictionary.

67. D.H. Hornig, U. Moser and B.E. Glatthaar. (1988) "Ascorbic Acid." In Modern Nutrition in Health and Disease, ed. M.E. Shils and V.R. Young, (Lea & Febiger, Philadelphia, PA), 420, 422, 407.

68. Hornig and Glatthaar, 420, 422, 407.

69. David M. Paige, M.D., M.P.H., Clinical Nutrition. (Washington, D.C.: C. V. Mosby Co., 1988), 571.

70. Tortora and Grabowski, 592, 595, 612, 615, 9, 604, 911.

71. Tortora and Grabowski, 592, 595, 612, 615, 9, 604, 911.

72. Tortora and Grabowski, 592, 595, 612, 615, 9, 604, 911.

73. Tortora and Grabowski, 592, 595, 612, 615, 9, 604, 911.

74. Recommended Dietary Allowances (RDA) 10th Ed., 174, 189, 255, 100.

75. Tortora and Grabowski, 592, 595, 612, 615, 9, 604, 911.

76. Tortora and Grabowski, 592, 595, 612, 615, 9, 604, 911.

77. Recommended Dietary Allowances (RDA) 10th Ed., 174, 189, 255, 100.

78. Tortora and Grabowski, 592, 595, 612, 615, 9, 604, 911.

79. Recommended Dietary Allowances (RDA) 10th Ed., 174, 189, 255, 100.

80. Recommended Dietary Allowances (RDA) 10th Ed., 174, 189, 255, 100.

81. Paige, 5, 557.

82. Tortora and Grabowski, 9.

83. The Bantam Medical Dictionary.

84. The Bantam Medical Dictionary.

85. Tortora and Grabowski, 43.

86. The Bantam Medical Dictionary.

87. Tortora and Grabowski, 79.

88. Suitor and Crowley, 36.

89. Suitor and Crowley, 37.

90. Tortora and Grabowski, 698-712, 699, 10, 683.

91. Tortora and Grabowski, 698-712, 699, 10, 683.

92. Quentinn Myrvik, "Nutrition and Immunology" in Modern Nutrition In Health and Disease (7th ed.), (Philadelphia: Lea and Febiger, 1988), 586, 588.

93. Tortora and Grabowski, 698-712, 699, 10, 683.

94. Myrvik, 586, 588.

95. Taber's Cyclopedic Medical Dictionary.

96. Louis V. Avioli, "Calcium and Phosphorus" in Modern Nutrition in Health and Disease, 142, 148.

97. Maurice E. Shils, "Magnesium" in Modern Nutrition in Health and Disease, 167-168, 173.

98. Suitor and Crowley, 52, 255, 46.

99. The Mosby Medical Encyclopedia, (Walter D. Glanze, Kenneth N. Anderson & Lois E. Anderson, eds.) (New York: Plume/Penguin Books, 1992).

100. Tortora and Grabowski, 683, 686, 689, 690, 705, 9.

101. The Mosby Medical Encyclopedia.

102. Tortora and Grabowski, 683, 686, 689, 690, 705, 9.

103. Tortora and Grabowski, 683, 686, 689, 690, 705, 9.

104. Tortora and Grabowski, 683, 686, 689, 690, 705, 9.

105. Davis and Sherer, 175.

106. Suitor, Carol West and Crowley, Merrily Forbes. Nutrition Principles and Application in Health Promotion (2nd ed.) Philadelphia: J.B. Lippincott Co. 1984.

107. Suitor, Carol West and Crowley, Merrily Forbes. Nutrition Principles and Application in Health Promotion (2nd ed.) Philadelphia: J.B. Lippincott Co. 1984.

108. Mahan, Kathleen L., and Escott-Stump, Sylvia. Krause's Food, Nutrition (9th ed.) W.B. Saunders Co. 1996. pp. 55, 111-112, 108, 69.

109. Robinson, Corinne H. Normal and Therapaeutic Nutrition, 17th ed. New York: Macmillan Publishing Co. 1990. pp. 173, 190.

110. Chaitow, Leon. N.D.,D.O., M.B.N.O.A Amino Acids in Therapy: A Guide to the Therapeutic Application of Protein Constituents. New York: Thorsons Pub. 1986. pp. 44, 45, 85.

111. Mahan, Kathleen L., and Escott-Stump, Sylvia. Krause's Food, Nutrition, (9th ed.) W.B. Saunders Co. 1996. pp. 55, 111-112, 108, 69.

112. Chaitow, Leon. N.D.,D.O., M.B.N.O.A Amino Acids in Therapy: A Guide to the Therapeutic Application of Protein Constituents. New York: Thorsons Pub. 1986, 44, 45, 85.

113. Chaitow, 44, 45, 85.

114. National Institute on Aging (NIA) - National Institutes of Health. Menopause, (Bethesda, MD, 1992), 1, 15, 20, 5, 27, 32.

115. National Institute on Aging (NIA) - National Institutes of Health. Menopause, (Bethesda, MD, 1992), 1, 15, 20, 5, 27, 32.

116. Tortora and Grabowski, 934, 45.

117. Tortora and Grabowski, 480, 485.

118. Paige, 333, 33.